2013

THE STATE OF FOOD AND AGRICULTURE

FOOD AND AGRICULTURE ORGANIZATION OF THE UNITED NATIONS
Rome, 2013

ISBN 978-92-5-107671-2 (print)
E-ISBN 978-92-5-107672-9 (PDF)

Contents

TABLES

BOXES

FIGURES

Foreword

As the world debates the Post-2015 Development Agenda, we must strive for nothing less than the eradication of hunger, food insecurity and malnutrition. The social and economic costs of malnutrition are unconscionably high, amounting to perhaps $US3.5 trillion per year or $US500 per person globally. Maternal and child malnutrition still impose a larger burden than overweight and obesity, although the latter is increasing even in developing regions. The challenge for the global community, therefore, is to continue fighting hunger and undernutrition while preventing or reversing the emergence of obesity.

This edition of *The State of Food and Agriculture: Food systems for better nutrition* makes the case that good nutrition begins with food and agriculture. Food systems around the world are diverse and changing rapidly. Food systems have become more industrial, commercial and global, unleashing processes of productivity growth, economic development and social transformation being felt around the world. These processes have profound implications for diets and nutritional outcomes.

Commercialization and specialization in agricultural production, processing and retailing have enhanced efficiency throughout the food system and increased the year-round availability and affordability of a diverse range of foods for most consumers in the world. At the same time, concerns are mounting about the sustainability of current consumption and production patterns, and their implications for nutritional outcomes.

Food systems must ensure that all people have access to a diverse range of nutritious foods and to the knowledge and information they need to make healthy choices. The contributions of food and agriculture to nutritional outcomes through production, prices and incomes are fundamental and must not be neglected, but food systems as a whole can contribute much more. This report identifies a number of specific actions that can be taken to improve the contribution of food systems to better nutrition. At the same time, reductions in food and nutrient losses throughout the food system can enhance both environmental sustainability and nutrition.

Food system strategies for nutrition are often contrasted with those that rely on medically based interventions such as vitamin and mineral supplements. Although food supplements can address specific dietary deficiencies, a nutritious diet ensures that people get the whole complex of nutrients they need and thus is the only approach that addresses all forms of malnutrition. What is more, food system strategies further recognize the social, psychological and cultural benefits that come from enjoying a variety of foods. Malnutrition is a complex problem that requires integrated action across sectors, but good nutrition must begin with food and agriculture. This report helps point the way.

José Graziano da Silva
FAO DIRECTOR-GENERAL

Acknowledgements

The State of Food and Agriculture 2013 was prepared by members of the Agricultural Development Economics Division (ESA) of FAO under the overall leadership of Kostas Stamoulis, Director; Keith Wiebe, Principal Officer; and Terri Raney, Senior Economist and Chief Editor. Additional guidance was provided by Barbara Burlingame, Principal Officer; James Garrett, Special Advisor; and Brian Thompson, Senior Officer of the Nutrition Division (ESN); David Hallam, Trade and Markets Division (EST); Jomo Kwame Sundaram, Assistant Director-General, Economic and Social Development Department (ADG-ES) and Daniel Gustafson, Deputy Director-General (Operations).

The research and writing team was led by André Croppenstedt and included Brian Carisma, Sarah Lowder, Terri Raney and Ellen Wielezynski (ESA); and James Garrett, Janice Meerman and Brian Thompson (ESN). The statistical annex was prepared by Brian Carisma under the supervision of Sarah Lowder, ESA. Additional inputs were provided by Aparajita Bijapurkar and Andrea Woolverton (ESA); Robert van Otterdijk, Rural Infrastructure and Agro-Industries Division (AGS); and Alexandre Meybeck, Agriculture and Consumer Protection Department (AGD).

The report was prepared in close collaboration with Janice Albert, Leslie Amoroso, Juliet Aphane, Ruth Charrondiere, Charlotte Dufour, Florence Egal, Anna Herforth, Gina Kennedy, Warren Lee, Ellen Muehlhoff, Valeria Menza, Martina Park and Holly Sedutto, all from (ESN); and *The State of Food and Agriculture* Focal Points: Daniela Battaglia, Animal Production and Health Division (AGA); Alison Hodder and Remi Kahane, Plant Production and Protection Division (AGP); David Kahan, Office of Knowledge Exchange, Research and Extension (OEK); Florence Tartanac and Anthony Bennett (AGS); Julien Custot and Jonathan Reeves, Climate, Energy and Tenure Division (NRC); Karel Callens, South-South and Resource Mobilization Division (TCS); Neil Marsland and Angela Hinrichs, Emergency and Rehabilitation Division (TCE); Maxim Lobovikov and Fred Kafeero, Forestry Economics, Policy and Products Division (FOE); Benoist Veillerette, Investment Centre Division (TCI); John Ryder, Fisheries and Aquaculture Policy and Economics Division (FIP); Eleonora Dupouy and David Sedik, Regional Office for Europe and Central Asia (REUT); Fatima Hachem, Regional Office for the Near East (FAORNE); David Dawe and Nomindelger Bayasgalanbat, Regional Office for Asia and the Pacific (FAORAP); Solomon Salcedo, Regional Office for Latin America and the Caribbean (FAORLC); and James Tefft, Regional Office for Africa (FAORAF). Additional inputs and reviews were provided by Jesús Barreiro-Hurlé, Juan Carlos García Cebolla, Maarten Immink, Joanna Jelensperger, Panagiotis Karfakis, Frank Mischler, Mark Smulders and Keith Wiebe (ESA); Terri Ballard, Ana Moltedo and Carlo Cafiero, Statistics Division (ESS); and Christina Rapone, Elisenda Estruch and Peter Wobst, Gender, Equity and Rural Employment Division (ESW).

External background papers and inputs were prepared by Christopher Barrett, Miguel Gómez, Erin Lentz, Dennis Miller, Per Pinstrup-Andersen, Katie Ricketts and Ross Welch (Cornell University); Bruce Traill (Reading University); Mario Mazzocchi (University of Bologna); Robert Mazur (Iowa State University); Action Contre la Faim/ACF-International; Save the Children (UK); Manan Chawla (Euromonitor); and Stephen Lim, Michael MacIntyre, Brittany Wurtz, Emily Carnahan and Greg Freedman (University of Washington).

The report benefited from external reviews and advice from many international experts: Francesco Branca, Mercedes de Onis, Marcella Wüstefeld and Gretchen Stevens, World Health Organization (WHO); Corinna Hawkes (World Cancer Research Fund International); Howarth Bouis and Yassir Islam (HarvestPlus); John McDermott, Agnes Quisumbing and Laurian Unnevehr, International Food Policy Research Institute

(IFPRI); Lynn Brown and Saskia de Pee, World Food Programme (WFP); Jennie Dey de Pryck, Mark Holderness and Harry Palmier, Global Forum on Agricultural Research (GFAR); Delia Grace, International Livestock Research Institute (ILRI); and Marie Arimond (University of California at Davis).

Michelle Kendrick, Economic and Social Development Department (ES), was responsible for publishing and project management. Paola Di Santo and Liliana Maldonado provided administrative support and Marco Mariani provided IT support throughout the process. We also gratefully acknowledge the support in organizing the technical workshop offered by David Hallam and organized by Jill Buscemi-Hicks, EST. Translations and printing services were provided by the FAO Meeting Programming and Documentation Service (CPAM). Graphic design and layout services were provided by Omar Bolbol and Flora Dicarlo.

Abbreviations and acronyms

BMI	body mass index
CONSEA	National Council for Food Security (Conselho Nacional de Segurança Alimentar e Nutricional)
DALY	disability-adjusted life year
EU	European Union
GDP	gross domestic product
HFP	Homestead Food Production (project)
IFPRI	International Food Policy Research Institute
MCLCP	Roundtable for Poverty Reduction (Mesa de Concertación para la Lucha Contra la Pobreza)
MDG	Millennium Development Goal
NGO	non-governmental organization
OECD	Organisation for Economic Co-operation and Development
OFSP	orange-fleshed sweet potato
R&D	research and development
REACH	Renewed Efforts Against Child Hunger and undernutrition
SUN	Scaling Up Nutrition
UN	United Nations
UNICEF	United Nations Children's Fund
UNSCN	United Nations Standing Committee on Nutrition
VAC	Vuon, Ao, Chuong (Crop farming, Aquaculture, Animal husbandry)
WFP	World Food Programme
WHO	World Health Organization
WIC	Supplemental Nutrition Program for Women, Infants, and Children (United States of America)

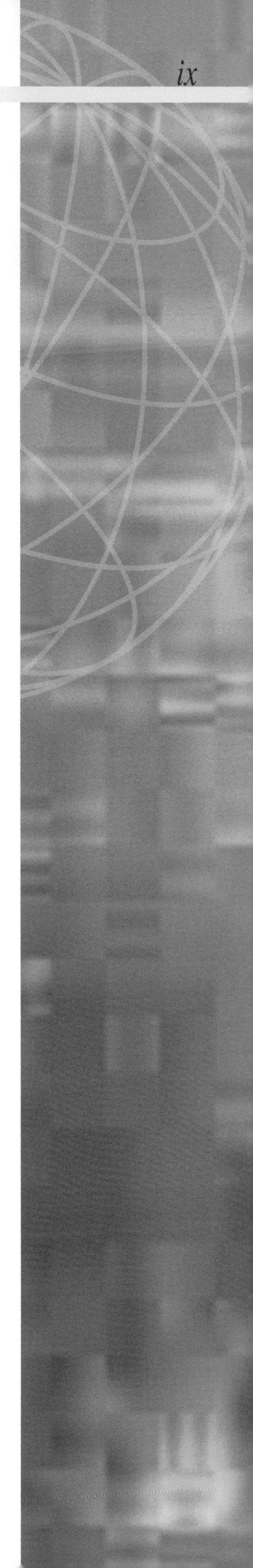

Executive summary

Malnutrition in all its forms – undernutrition, micronutrient deficiencies, and overweight and obesity – imposes unacceptably high economic and social costs on countries at all income levels. *The State of Food and Agriculture 2013: Food systems for better nutrition* argues that improving nutrition and reducing these costs must begin with food and agriculture. The traditional role of agriculture in producing food and generating income is fundamental, but agriculture and the entire food system – from inputs and production, through processing, storage, transport and retailing, to consumption – can contribute much more to the eradication of malnutrition.

Malnutrition imposes high costs on society

FAO's most recent estimates indicate that 12.5 percent of the world's population (868 million people) are undernourished in terms of energy intake, yet these figures represent only a fraction of the global burden of malnutrition. An estimated 26 percent of the world's children are stunted, 2 billion people suffer from one or more micronutrient deficiencies and 1.4 billion people are overweight, of whom 500 million are obese. Most countries are burdened by multiple types of malnutrition, which may coexist within the same country, household or individual.

The social cost of malnutrition, measured by the "disability-adjusted life years" lost to child and maternal malnutrition and to overweight and obesity, are very high. Beyond the social cost, the cost to the global economy caused by malnutrition, as a result of lost productivity and direct health care costs, could account for as much as 5 percent of global gross domestic product (GDP), equivalent to US$3.5 trillion per year or US$500 per person. The costs of undernutrition and micronutrient deficiencies are estimated at 2–3 percent of global GDP, equivalent to US$1.4–2.1 trillion per year. Although no global estimates of the economic costs of overweight and obesity exist, the cumulative cost of all non-communicable diseases, for which overweight and obesity are leading risk factors, were estimated to be about US$1.4 trillion in 2010.

Child and maternal malnutrition – in particular child underweight, child micronutrient deficiencies and poor breastfeeding practices – impose by far the largest nutrition-related health burden at the global level, responsible for almost twice the social costs of adult overweight and obesity. The social burden due to child and maternal malnutrition has declined almost by half during the last two decades, while that due to overweight and obesity has almost doubled, yet the former remains by far the greater problem, especially in low-income countries. Undernutrition and micronutrient deficiencies must therefore continue to be the highest nutrition priority for the global community in the immediate future. The challenge for policy-makers is how to address these problems while at the same time avoiding or reversing the emergence of overweight and obesity. This challenge is significant, but the returns are high: investing in the reduction of micronutrient deficiencies, for example, would result in better health, fewer child deaths and increased future earnings, with a benefit-to-cost ratio of almost 13 to 1.

Addressing malnutrition requires integrated action across sectors

The immediate causes of malnutrition are complex and multidimensional. They include inadequate availability of and access to safe, diverse, nutritious food; lack of access to clean water, sanitation and health care; and inappropriate child feeding and adult dietary choices. The root causes of malnutrition are even more complex and encompass the broader economic, social, political, cultural and physical environment. Addressing malnutrition, therefore, requires integrated action and complementary interventions in agriculture and the food system in general, in public health and education, as well as in

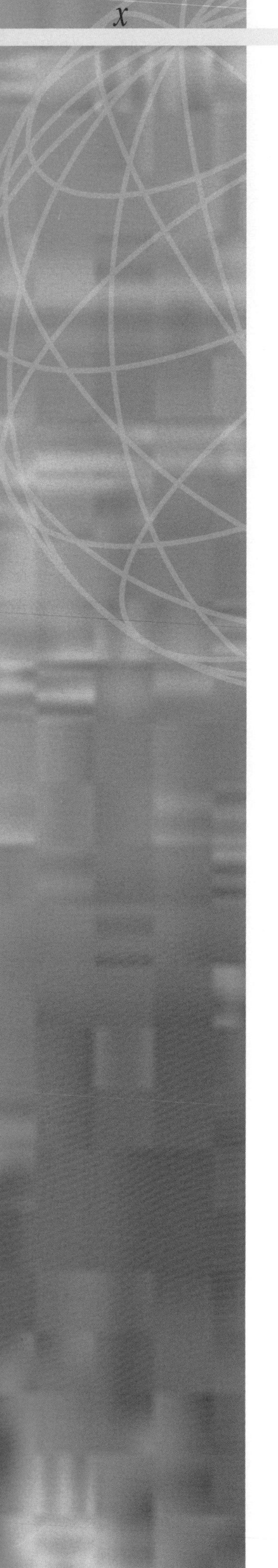

broader policy domains. Because the necessary interventions cut across the portfolios of several government institutions, high-level political support is required to motivate the necessary coordination across sectors.

Better nutrition depends on every aspect of the food system

Food systems encompass all the people, institutions and processes by which agricultural products are produced, processed and brought to consumers. They also include the public officials, civil society organizations, researchers and development practitioners who design the policies, regulations, programmes and projects that shape food and agriculture.

Every aspect of the food system influences the availability and accessibility of diverse, nutritious foods and thus the ability of consumers to choose healthy diets. But the linkages from the food system to nutritional outcomes are often indirect – mediated through incomes, prices, knowledge and other factors. What is more, food system policies and interventions are rarely designed with nutrition as their primary objective, so impacts can be difficult to trace and researchers sometimes conclude that food system interventions are ineffective in reducing malnutrition. In contrast, medical interventions such as vitamin supplements can address specific nutrient deficiencies and their impacts are more easily observed, but they cannot fully substitute for the broader nutritional benefits offered by a well-functioning food system. Every aspect of the food system must align to support good nutrition; any single intervention in isolation is therefore unlikely to have a significant impact within such a complex system. Interventions that consider food systems as a whole are more likely to achieve positive nutritional outcomes.

Nutrition transition is driven by food system transformation

Economic and social development lead to the gradual transformation of agriculture, characterized by rising labour productivity, declining shares of population working in agriculture and rising urbanization. New modes of transportation, leisure, employment and work within the home cause people to lead more sedentary lifestyles and to demand more convenient foods. These changes in activity and dietary patterns are part of a "nutrition transition" in which households and countries may simultaneously face the emerging challenge of overweight, obesity and related non-communicable diseases while continuing to deal with undernutrition and micronutrient deficiencies. The complexity and rapidly changing nature of both the malnutrition situation and food systems in individual countries mean that policies and interventions need to be context-specific.

Agricultural productivity growth contributes to nutrition but must do more

Agricultural productivity growth contributes to better nutrition through raising incomes, especially in countries where the sector accounts for a large share of the economy and employment, and by reducing the cost of food for all consumers. It is, however, important to realize that the impact of agricultural productivity growth is slow and may not be sufficient to cause a rapid reduction in malnutrition.

Maintaining the momentum of growth in agricultural productivity will remain crucial in the coming decades as production of basic staple foods needs to increase by 60 percent if it is to meet expected demand growth. Beyond staple foods, healthy diets are diverse, containing a balanced and adequate combination of energy, fat and protein, as well as micronutrients. Agricultural research and development priorities must be made more nutrition-sensitive, with a stronger focus on nutrient-dense foods such as fruits, vegetables, legumes and animal-source foods. Greater efforts must be directed towards interventions that diversify smallholder production, such as integrated farming systems. Efforts to raise the micronutrient content of staples directly through biofortification are particularly promising. Agricultural interventions are generally more effective when combined with nutrition education and implemented with sensitivity to gender roles.

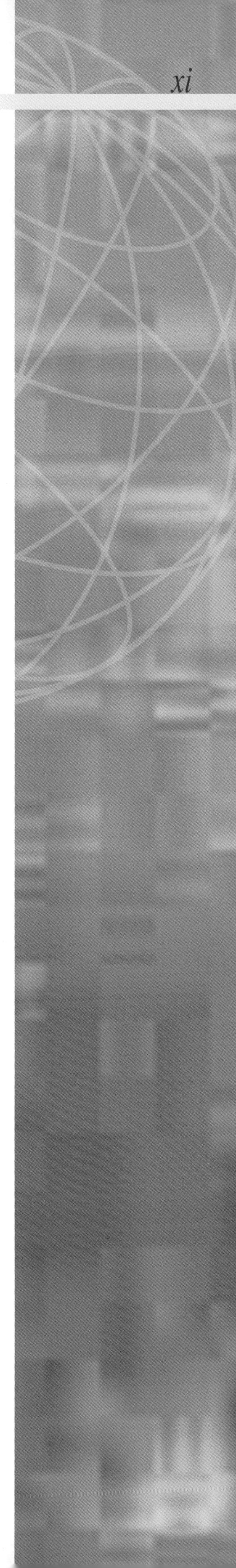

Supply chains offer risks and opportunities for better nutrition

Traditional and modern food systems coexist and evolve as economies grow and urbanization increases. Modern supply chains entail vertical integration of storage, distribution and retailing and offer efficiency gains that can yield lower prices for consumers and higher incomes for farmers. They typically carry a wide variety of nutritious foods year-round, but also sell more highly processed packaged foods, which can contribute to overweight and obesity when consumed in excess. Modern food processing and distribution also offer new opportunities for the use of fortified foods, which can make important contributions to nutrition.

Although supermarkets are spreading rapidly in low-income countries, most poor consumers in rural and urban areas still purchase most of their food through traditional food distribution networks. These traditional outlets are the primary channel for nutrient-rich foods such as fruits, vegetables and livestock products, although they increasingly carry processed and packaged foods. The use of traditional retail outlets for distributing fortified foods such as iodized salt is another proven strategy for improving nutritional outcomes.

Improved sanitation, food handling, and storage technologies in traditional food systems could boost efficiency and improve the safety and nutritional quality of foods. Reducing food and nutrient losses and waste throughout food systems could make important contributions to better nutrition and relieve pressure on productive resources.

Consumer choices determine nutritional outcomes and sustainability

Making systems more nutrition-enhancing so that food is available, accessible, diverse and nutritious is key, but so is the need to help consumers make healthy dietary choices. Promoting behaviour change through nutrition education and information campaigns within a supportive environment that also addresses household sanitation and appropriate complementary foods has proved effective. Even in locations where undernutrition and micronutrient deficiencies persist as the primary problems, a forward-looking approach that can prevent a rise in overweight and obesity is necessary, especially in the long run. Behaviour change can also reduce food waste and contribute to the sustainable use of resources.

Institutional and policy environment for nutrition

Progress has been made: in some countries malnutrition has been significantly reduced over recent decades. But progress has been uneven and there is a pressing need to make better use of the food system for better nutrition. The complexity of malnutrition and its underlying causes means that a multistakeholder and multisectoral approach will be most effective.

Such an approach requires better governance, based on sound data, a common vision and political leadership to be able to plan, coordinate and foster the necessary collaboration across and within sectors.

Key messages of the report

- **Malnutrition in all its forms imposes unacceptably high costs on society in human and economic terms.** The costs associated with undernutrition and micronutrient deficiencies are higher than those associated with overweight and obesity, although the latter are rising rapidly even in low- and middle-income countries.
- **Addressing malnutrition requires a multisectoral approach that includes complementary interventions in food systems, public health and education.** This approach also facilitates the pursuit of multiple objectives, including better nutrition, gender equality and environmental sustainability.
- **Within a multisectoral approach, food systems offer many opportunities for interventions leading to improved diets and better nutrition.** Some of these interventions have the primary purpose of enhancing nutrition. Other

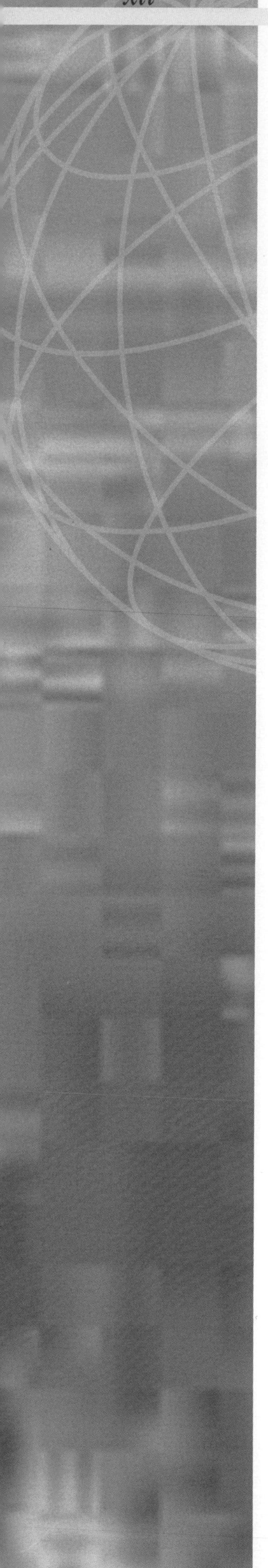

interventions in food systems, and in the general economic, social or political environment, may affect nutrition even though this is not their primary objective.

- **Agricultural production and productivity growth remain essential for better nutrition, but more can be done.** Agricultural research must continue to enhance productivity, while paying greater attention to nutrient-dense foods such as fruits, vegetables, legumes and animal products and to more sustainable production systems. Production interventions are more effective when they are sensitive to gender roles and combined with nutrition education.
- **Both traditional and modern supply chains offer risks and opportunities for achieving better nutrition and more sustainable food systems.** Improvements in traditional supply chains can help reduce losses, lower prices and increase diversity of choice for lower-income households. The growth of modern retailing and food processing can facilitate the use of fortification to combat malnutrition, but the increased availability of highly processed, packaged goods may contribute to overweight and obesity.
- **Consumers ultimately determine what they eat and therefore what the food system produces.** But governments, international organizations, the private sector and civil society can all help consumers make healthier decisions, reduce waste and contribute to the sustainable use of resources, by providing clear, accurate information and ensuring access to diverse and nutritious foods.
- **Better governance of food systems at all levels, facilitated by high-level political support, is needed to build a common vision, to support evidence-based policies, and to promote effective coordination and collaboration through integrated, multisectoral action.**

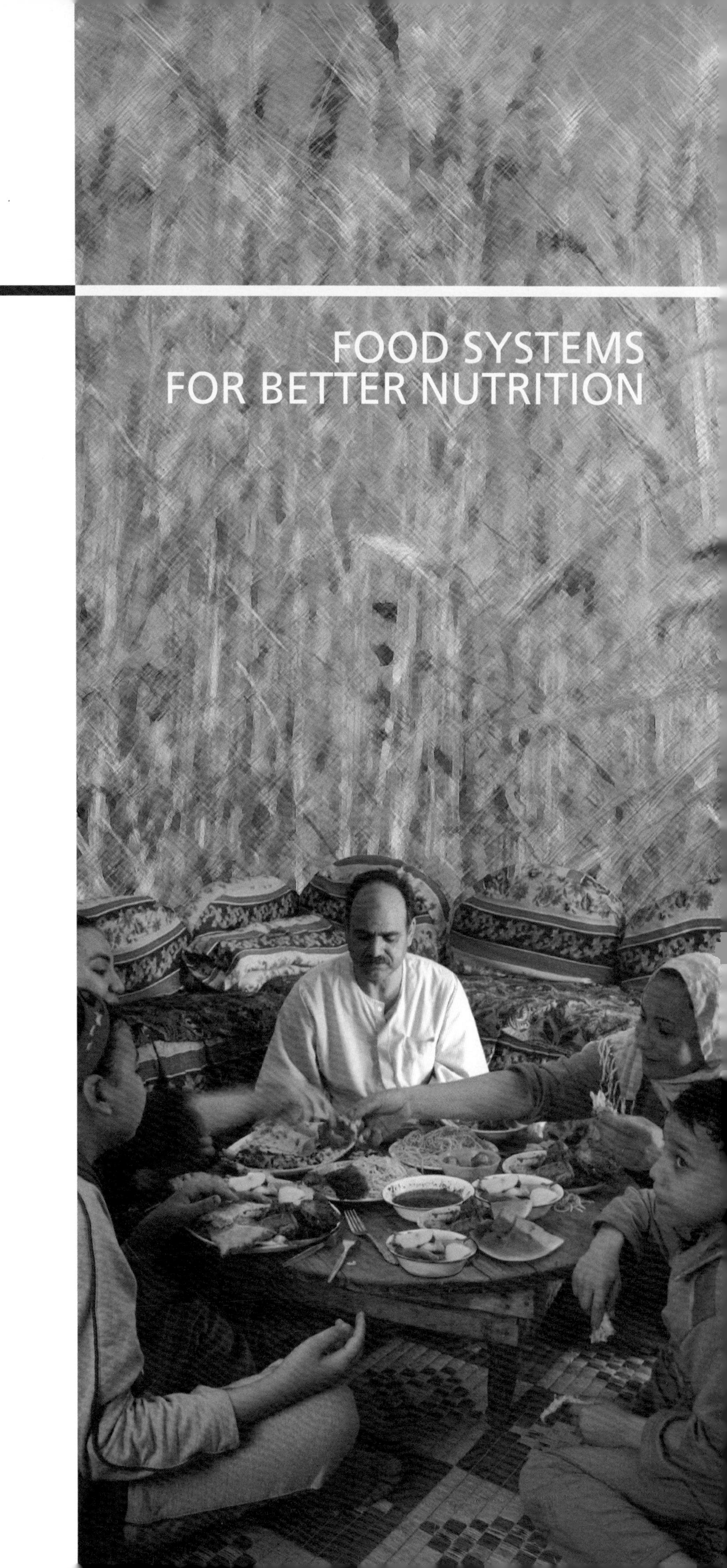

FOOD SYSTEMS FOR BETTER NUTRITION

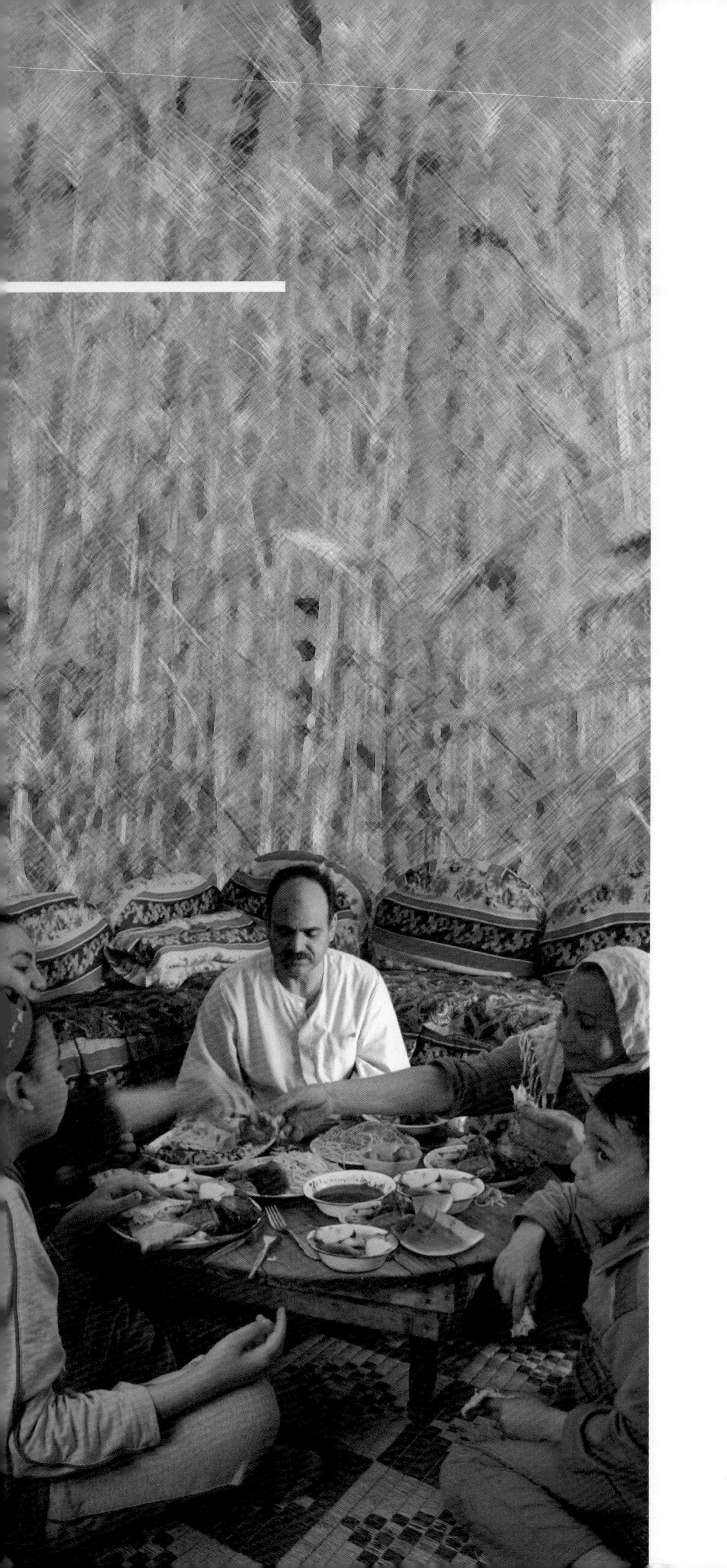

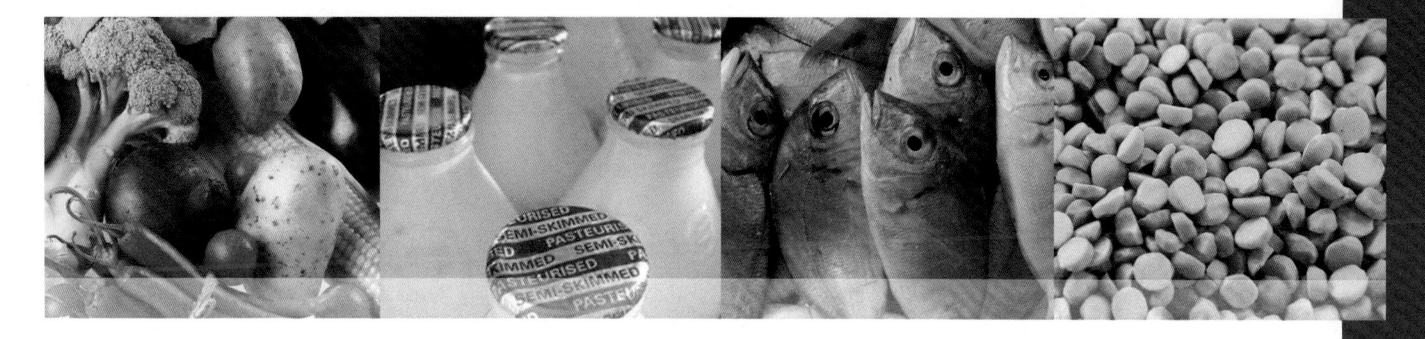

1. The role of food systems in nutrition

Malnutrition in all its forms[1] – undernutrition, micronutrient deficiencies, and overweight and obesity – imposes high economic and social costs on countries at all income levels. This edition of *The State of Food and Agriculture* makes the case that food systems[2] – from agricultural inputs and production; through processing, marketing and retailing, to consumption – can promote more nutritious and sustainable diets for everyone.

The first edition of *The State of Food and Agriculture*, published in 1947, reported that about half of the world's population was chronically malnourished, considered at that time primarily in terms of inadequate energy consumption. FAO's latest estimates indicate that the proportion of the world's population suffering from undernourishment has declined to 12.5 percent; this is a remarkable achievement, yet 868 million people remain undernourished in terms of energy consumption and an estimated 2 billion people suffer from one or more micronutrient deficiencies (FAO, IFAD and WFP, 2012). Twenty-six percent of all children under the age of five are stunted and 31 percent suffer from vitamin A deficiency, while an estimated 1.4 billion people are overweight, of whom 500 million are obese (WHO, 2013a).

Food systems around the world are diverse and changing rapidly, with profound implications for diets and nutritional outcomes. Since 1947, food systems have become more industrial, commercial and global. The substitution of mechanical, chemical and biological technologies for land and labour in agricultural production has unleashed processes of productivity growth, economic development and social transformation that are being felt around the world. Commercialization and specialization in agricultural production, processing and retailing have enhanced efficiency throughout the food system and increased the year-round availability and affordability of a diverse range of foods for most consumers in the world. At the same time, concerns are mounting about the sustainability of current consumption and production patterns, and their implications for nutritional outcomes (Box 1).

While the nature and causes of malnutrition are complex, the common denominator among all types of malnutrition is a nutritionally inappropriate diet. The potential of food systems to contribute to the eradication of malnutrition goes beyond the fundamental role of agriculture in producing food and generating income. Of course, addressing malnutrition requires interventions not only in the food system, but also in the health, sanitation, education and other sectors. Integrated actions are needed across the health, education and agriculture sectors.

[1] Malnutrition is defined in detail at the start of Chapter 2.
[2] Food systems encompass the entire range of activities involved in the production, processing, marketing, consumption and disposal of goods that originate from agriculture, forestry or fisheries, including the inputs needed and the outputs generated at each of these steps. Food systems also involve the people and institutions that initiate or inhibit change in the system as well as the socio-political, economic and technological environment in which these activities take place. Adapted from FAO (2012a).

BOX 1
Sustainable production and consumption

The importance of managing agricultural systems in a way that ensures the sustainability of natural resource use is already well established. Most of the focus has been on the production side, where the emphasis is on sustainable intensification that can close yield and productivity gaps in underperforming systems while reducing the negative and enhancing the positive environmental impacts of agriculture (FAO, 2011a). This focus on sustainable production continues to be of great importance for people whose consumption levels are insufficient to sustain a healthy and active life. But it is also recognized that the costs and benefits of a sustainable system must also be reflected in decisions made by consumers and producers, as well as policy-makers (FAO, 2012b).

Sustainable consumption is captured by the concept of sustainable diets, that is: "those diets with low environmental impacts which contribute to food and nutrition security and to healthy life for present and future generations. Sustainable diets are protective and respectful of biodiversity and ecosystems, culturally acceptable, accessible, economically fair and affordable; nutritionally adequate, safe and healthy; while optimizing natural and human resources" (Burlingame and Dernini, 2012, p. 7).

Sustainable diets imply a change in dietary preferences to reduce overconsumption and a shift to nutritious diets with lower environmental footprints. They also mean a reduction of losses and waste throughout the food system. Ultimately, the aim of a successful transition to healthier and sustainable diets is for people and the ecosystem to be healthier. Such profound changes are likely to require significant changes in the food systems themselves.

For the full values of natural resources and the environment to be paid by consumers and producers, these values should be embedded in the planning, institutions, technologies and value chains. There is a need to build consumer awareness through information and education, to remove subsidies that encourage unsustainable resource use and to use differential taxation to reflect the full value of natural resources. The many issues to be addressed include the role of livestock and fish in diets, the role of local and traded foods and the link between food and non-food agricultural products. Many of these issues are highly controversial because their implications extend beyond production and consumption to trade, and so they require dialogue and agreement among international stakeholders. Not all changes are controversial, however, for example the need to reduce losses and waste. Regardless, a transition to sustainable diets will have significant implications for producers, the food industry, consumers, land use and trade rules. These challenges require inclusive and evidence-based governance mechanisms that can address the many needs and trade-offs involved. There is currently little agreement either nationally or internationally on practical ways to implement the concept of sustainable diets (UNEP, 2012).

Why is nutrition important?

Good nutrition is the foundation for human health and well-being, physical and cognitive development, and economic productivity. Nutritional status is a critical indicator of overall human and economic development, and good nutritional status is an essential social benefit in its own right. As an input to social and economic development, good nutrition is the key to breaking intergenerational cycles of poverty, because good maternal nutrition produces healthier children, who grow into healthier adults. Good nutrition reduces disease and raises labour productivity and incomes, including of people working in agriculture.

Global losses in economic productivity due to undernutrition and micronutrient deficiencies have been estimated at more than 10 percent of lifetime earnings and 2–3 percent of global gross domestic product (GDP) (World Bank, 2006a). The latter figure translates into a global cost of US$1.4–2.1 trillion.

At the same time, obesity is associated with lower labour productivity and higher medical costs arising from associated non-communicable chronic diseases, such as diabetes and heart disease (WHO, 2011a). A recent study estimates a cumulative output loss due to non-communicable diseases, for which overweight and obesity are key risk factors, of US$47 trillion over the next two decades; on an annual basis and assuming a 5 percent rate of inflation, this is equivalent to about US$1.4 trillion in 2010 (Bloom *et al.*, 2011).

No comprehensive global estimates exist for the productivity losses and health costs associated with all types of malnutrition and related diseases. The partial estimates reported above can be summed to provide a rough estimate of global costs. This approach suggests that malnutrition in all its forms may impose a cost of US$2.8–3.5 trillion, equivalent to 4–5 percent of global GDP, or US$400–500 per person.[3]

Investments in reducing micronutrient deficiencies would have high pay-offs. Deficiencies in micronutrients can slow intellectual and physical growth among children, reduce adult labour productivity and lead to disease, premature death and increased maternal mortality (UNICEF and The Micronutrient Initiative, 2004; Micronutrient Initiative, 2009). No global estimates of the economic costs of micronutrient deficiencies exist; however, addressing such deficiencies and their consequences is one of the most valuable investments society can make. The Copenhagen Consensus project, for example, which brings together world experts to consider the most cost-effective solutions to leading world problems, highlighted the provision of micronutrients as a cost-effective means to tackle the problem of malnutrition. Research showed that investing US$1.2 billion annually in micronutrient supplements, food fortification and biofortification of staple crops for five years would generate annual benefits of US$15.3 billion, a benefit-to-cost ratio of almost 13 to 1, and would result in better health, fewer deaths and increased future earnings (Micronutrient Initiative, 2009).

Malnutrition – whether undernutrition, micronutrient deficiencies or overweight and obesity – is caused by a complex interplay of economic, social, environmental and behavioural factors that prevent people from consuming and fully benefiting from healthy diets. The most immediate causes of undernutrition and micronutrient deficiencies are inadequate dietary intake and infectious disease. Inadequate dietary intake weakens the immune system and increases susceptibility to disease; infectious disease, in turn, increases nutrient requirements and further weakens the immune system. There are three underlying causes of this vicious cycle: (i) lack of availability or access to food (food insecurity); (ii) poor health mediated by poor water and sanitation and inadequate health services; and (iii), for children, poor maternal and child-care practices, including inadequate breastfeeding and nutritious complementary feeding and, for adults, poor food choices. Of course, deeper forces of social and economic underdevelopment and inequality often underpin these problems.

The most immediate cause of overweight and obesity is overconsumption of energy relative to physical requirements, yet nutritionists have long recognized that this does not explain why some people consume more than they need. The rapid increase in the prevalence of overweight and obesity in recent decades has prompted many explanations, including genetic predisposition, viral or bacteriological infections that alter energy requirements, endocrine disruptors, the use of certain pharmaceutical products, and social and economic factors that encourage overconsumption (Greenway, 2006; Keith *et al.*, 2006).[4] Changes in the food system since the mid-twentieth century have also been implicated, including lower real prices of food, changes in relative prices of different types of food and increased availability of highly processed, energy-dense, micronutrient-poor foods (Rosenheck, 2008; Popkin, Adair and Ng, 2012).

[3] US$1.4–2.1 trillion for undernutrition and micronutrient deficiencies plus US$1.4 trillion for non-communicable diseases equals US$2.8–3.5 trillion.

[4] Some of these are theories that have not yet been empirically substantiated.

Why focus on food systems to address malnutrition?

Nutritional outcomes depend on many factors, but food systems and the policies and institutions that shape them are a fundamental part of the equation. A common denominator across all types of malnutrition is the appropriateness of the diets consumed. At the most basic level, food systems determine the quantity, quality, diversity and nutritional content of the foods available for consumption.

Agricultural production and trade policies and public investments in research and development (R&D) and in infrastructure are some of the factors that influence the supply of different types of foods. Income, culture and education, among other factors, influence consumers' tastes and preferences, which, together with relative prices, determine the demand for different foods. Demand, in turn, influences production as well as processing and marketing decisions throughout the food system, in a continuous cycle of feed-back loops. The food system thus determines whether the food people need for good nutrition is available, affordable, acceptable and of adequate quantity and quality.

The principle of shaping food and agricultural systems to improve nutrition is founded and builds on a food-based approach. Food-based interventions recognize the central place of food and diets in improving nutrition. They are often contrasted with strategies that rely on medically based interventions such as vitamin and mineral supplements. Although food supplements can address specific dietary deficiencies, a nutritious diet (meaning consumption of a variety of safe foods of sufficient quantity and quality in the appropriate combinations) ensures that people obtain not only the specific macro- or micronutrients present in the supplement but the whole complex of energy, nutrients and fibre that they need. These components of a nutritious diet may interact in ways that are important for good nutrition and health but are not yet fully understood.

A food-based approach further recognizes the multiple benefits (nutritional, physiological, mental, social and cultural) that come from enjoying a variety of foods. Creating a strong nutrition-enhancing food system is arguably the most practical, convenient and sustainable way to address malnutrition, as food choices and consumption patterns ultimately become integrated into the lifestyle of the individual (FAO, 2010).

In addressing malnutrition, considering the entire food system provides a framework in which to determine, design and implement food-based interventions to improve nutrition. Shaping food systems so they are more likely to lead to better diets and nutritional outcomes requires an understanding of the different elements of the system, potential entry points to leverage the system for nutrition and the factors that shape the choices of the different actors in the system. In addition, in today's world, analyses and actions must also demonstrate close attention to questions of environmental sustainability.

Changes and challenges in food systems of today

Analyses and actions to shape food systems for better nutrition must take into account the fact that there is no single food system but rather a multiplicity of systems with characteristics that vary, for example, with incomes, livelihoods and urbanization. Even these multiple systems are in a process of constant change. Trends in economies and societies, from local to global level, are changing the ways that people produce, process and acquire food.

In developing countries as well as more industrialized countries, food supply chains are transforming in many ways. For some consumers and some products, the supply chain is lengthening. Most people today, even the poorest smallholders in remote rural areas, rely on markets for at least part of their consumption needs. They may buy surpluses from local producers or, in the case of processed foods like biscuits or pasta, from processors in far-away cities or countries. The distance between consumer and producer may grow for such products as transportation networks improve and trade increases.

At the same time, for people in urban areas even in developing countries, the supply chain may be shortening or lengthening depending on the product. Consumers may shop directly at farmers' markets, especially for fresh fruits and vegetables, or in traditional wet markets for meat products. Wholesalers, often with strong links to modern retail chains, may buy staple products directly from producers, bypassing traditional local brokers (Reardon and Minten, 2011). Meanwhile, supply chains for some products may be becoming more complex, with additional transformation of products by processors and distributors.

The kinds of food being demanded are also changing. New technologies are altering modes of transportation, leisure, employment and work within the home (Popkin, Adair and Ng, 2012). Increasingly, urban lifestyles lead consumers to demand more convenience, because they have less time available or simply wish to devote less time to food production, acquisition and preparation.

Urbanization also provides economies of scale for markets, resulting in lower transport costs and markets that are generally closer to home. Combined with generally higher incomes for urban dwellers, these changes widen the selection of products available. Although the diversity of choice leads to higher consumption of animal-source foods and fruits and vegetables, increases in consumption of processed foods also lead to higher intakes of fats, sugars and salt. With higher energy intakes and lower energy expenditure, urban dwellers incur a higher risk of overweight and obesity than rural dwellers. These changes in purchasing and consumption patterns are occurring in smaller cities and towns as well as the largest cities. Through their research and marketing efforts, food companies, of course, are shaping as well as responding to these demands.

These changes in activity and dietary patterns in developing countries are part of a "nutrition transition" in which countries simultaneously face not only the emerging challenge of rising levels of overweight and obesity and related non-communicable diseases but continue to deal with problems of undernutrition and micronutrient deficiencies (Bray and Popkin, 1998). This transition corresponds closely to rises in income and the structural transformation of the food system, as seen primarily in industrialized and middle-income countries. Popkin, Adair and Ng (2012, p. 3) describe this phenomenon as "the primary mismatch between human biology and modern society". All this suggests that the nature of the nutrition problem and its solutions may differ according to location and type of engagement with the food system.

Food systems and nutrition opportunities

The structure of food systems is central to determining how those systems interact with other causal factors and influence nutritional outcomes. Awareness of these characteristics and the key actors who shape food systems will help identify where to intervene and what to do to create systems that help achieve good nutrition.

The multiple links between food systems and nutrition offer many opportunities to shape food systems in such a way that they can promote better nutrition. Figure 1 provides a schematic overview of the elements of food systems and the broader economic, social, cultural and physical environment within which they operate. It highlights opportunities for improving nutritional outcomes and identifies appropriate policy tools.

The first column outlines the elements of a food system, in three broad categories:

- production "up to the farm gate";
- post-harvest supply chain "from the farm gate to retailer";
- consumers.

The middle column lists examples of potential interventions that are targeted specifically at improving nutrition – "opportunities", that is, to shape the system. The third column notes some policy tools related primarily to food, agriculture and rural development that can influence the system. The outer ring illustrates the broader context, which can also be made more "nutrition-sensitive", for example by giving higher priority to nutrition within national development strategies and considering the nutrition implications of broader macroeconomic policies, the status of women and environmental sustainability.

The phases from production to consumption are depicted in a linear representation, but the interactions among the various actors and the flows of their influence are not. Demand by consumers or processors, for example, can affect what is produced, and multiple stakeholders can exert influences on the system and the policy context at different

FIGURE 1
Food system interventions for better nutrition

Policy environment and development priorities

Economic, social, cultural and physical environment

Gender roles and environmental sustainability

FOOD SYSTEM ELEMENTS	NUTRITION OPPORTUNITIES	POLICY TOOLS
Production "up to the farm gate" (R&D, inputs, production, farm management)	• Sustainable intensification of production • Nutrition-promoting farming systems, agronomic practices and crops - Micronutrient fertilizers - Biofortified crops - Integrated farming systems, including fisheries and forestry - Crop and livestock diversification • Stability for food security and nutrition - Grain reserves and storage - Crop and livestock insurance • Nutrition education - School and home gardens • Nutrient preserving on-farm storage	• Food and agricultural policies to promote availability, affordability, diversity and quality • Nutrition-oriented agricultural research on crops, livestock and production systems • Promotion of school and home gardens
Post-harvest supply chain "from the farm gate to retailer" (marketing, storage, trade, processing, retailing)	• Nutrient-preserving processing, packaging, transport and storage • Reduced waste and increased technical and economic efficiency • Food fortification • Reformulation for better nutrition (e.g. elimination of trans fats) • Food safety	• Regulation and taxation to promote efficiency, safety, quality, diversity • Research and promotion of innovation in product formulation, processing and transport
Consumers (advertising, labelling, education, safety nets)	• Nutrition information and health claims • Product labelling • Consumer education • Social protection for food security and nutrition - General food assistance programmes and subsidies - Targeted food assistance (prenatal, children, elderly, etc.)	• Food assistance programmes • Food price incentives • Nutrition regulations • Nutrition education and information campaigns

AVAILABLE, ACCESSIBLE, DIVERSE, NUTRITIOUS FOODS

Health, food safety, education, sanitation and infrastructure

Source: FAO.

points and in different ways. Considering the entire food system is thus more complex and integrated than a simple commodity value-chain approach, which is likely to focus on the technical aspects of various stages of the chain and usually considers only one crop or product at a time.

Addressing the entire food system implies appreciating and working with all the different stakeholders who affect the system. These include all people – primarily private individuals and companies – who produce, store, process, market and consume food, as well as the public officials, civil society organizations, researchers and development practitioners who design the policies, regulations, programmes and projects that shape the system.

Figure 1 should be understood as a stylized representation of the many diverse and dynamic food systems that exist in the world. The nature of the food system in a given location can guide the choice of interventions to take advantage of nutrition opportunities. For example, in a subsistence-based agricultural system, interventions aimed directly at improving the nutritional content of crops for own consumption would be promising. In urban areas where the food system is almost entirely commercial, interventions in processing and retailing could be more effective in shaping the system to support better nutrition. Many developing countries have food systems that exhibit a mix of characteristics.

Promoting nutrition-specific and nutrition-sensitive actions

Many of the nutrition opportunities highlighted in Figure 1 and in later chapters of this report are nutrition-specific. They are pursued with the primary purpose of making the system more attuned to producing good nutritional outcomes. For example, the principal impetus in developing biofortified crops is to improve nutrition. At the same time, these crops may also be more disease-resistant and better adapted to grow in micronutrient-deficient soils. They may improve nutrition but also produce higher crop yields and increase producer incomes – a win for both consumers and producers (Harvest Plus, 2011).

Other interventions, particularly those that improve the general economic, social or political environment, may not be specifically designed to improve nutrition but will almost certainly have a positive effect. Examples of these "nutrition-sensitive actions" include policies that increase agricultural productivity (which can raise producer incomes, lower the cost of food for consumers and allow producers and consumers to increase expenditures on more adequate, diverse diets) or that improve the social status of women (and so can lead to increased expenditures on health, education and food, which are all key inputs into better nutrition).

Similarly, in a nutrition-sensitive environment, governments or companies may simply take into account the potential impacts of their actions on nutrition and seek to leverage any positive effects or mitigate any negative ones. For instance, the introduction of new crops might lead to higher productivity and household incomes, but might also make higher demands on women's labour. This could lead to negative impacts on child care that a nutrition-sensitive approach would address. In sum, the difference in primary purpose (often driven by the context of the opportunity) is what distinguishes nutrition-specific interventions from ones that are nutrition-sensitive. Although the overall objective may be to create a nutrition-sensitive food system, interventions in agriculture and food systems may be both nutrition-specific and nutrition-sensitive.

Cross-cutting issues in nutrition-sensitive food systems

Many interventions are specific to a particular part of the food system, but there are some issues that nearly all interventions need to address. For example, gender issues are always relevant because men and women, who participate in every part of the food system, have different roles and therefore will be affected differently by any intervention aimed at making food systems more nutrition-sensitive. Similarly, concerns related to environmental sustainability touch every aspect of the food system and have fundamental implications for nutrition. Diets that are diverse and environmentally sustainable are the foundation for better nutritional outcomes for everyone and should be a long-term goal for all food systems.

Gender roles for better nutritional outcomes

Men and women typically play differentiated roles in food systems and within the household, although these differences vary widely by region and are changing rapidly (FAO, 2011b). Women make important and growing contributions to food production, processing, marketing and retailing, and other parts of the food system. Within the household, women traditionally bear the primary responsibility for preparing meals and caring for children and other family members, although men are assuming more responsibilities for these roles in many societies. Gender differences in the rights, resources and responsibilities – particularly resources necessary for achieving food and nutrition security for and within the household and responsibilities for food provisioning and caretaking – often impede the achievement of household food and nutrition security.

Gender-sensitive interventions can improve nutritional outcomes by recognizing women's role in nutrition through agricultural production, food provision and child care and by promoting gender equality throughout the system, including in some cases by increasing the participation of men in household maintenance, food preparation and child care. In agriculture, technologies that enhance the labour productivity of rural women (such as better farm tools, water provision, modern energy services and household food preparation) can free their time for other activities. For example, a study from India demonstrated that women who used a groundnut decorticator were able to process around 14 times more groundnuts and used significantly less physical effort than those doing so by hand. Similarly, a new hand tool designed for making ridges for vegetable crops allowed women to double the number of rows finished in one hour (Singh, Puna Ji Gite and Agarwal, 2006). Such innovations in technology may open up opportunities for women to earn higher incomes or to use their time (and increased income) for added attention to the family.

Women are also active in other parts of the food system, including food marketing and processing. For example, in Latin America and the Caribbean and in Africa, women dominate employment in many of the high-value agricultural commodity chains. Although new jobs in export-oriented agro-industries may not employ men and women on equal terms, they often provide better opportunities for women than exist within the confines of traditional agriculture (FAO, 2011b).

Raising women's incomes has important implications for nutritional outcomes, because women still play a central role in shaping household food consumption patterns. Women who earn more income have stronger bargaining power within the household. This enables them to exert more influence over decisions regarding consumption, investment and production, which results in better nutrition, health and education outcomes for children (Smith *et al.*, 2003; Quisumbing, 2003; FAO, 2011b; Duflo, 2012; World Bank, 2011).

Sustainable food systems

The importance of managing the agriculture system in a way that is conducive to the health of the ecosystem is already well established. To date, most of the focus has been on the production side, with the emphasis on sustainable intensification that can close yield and productivity gaps in underperforming systems (FAO, 2011c). This continues to be of great importance, especially for poor farmers. Yet improving the sustainability of food systems is equally important. Environmentally and economically sustainable production is important for the well-being of current and future generations. Reductions in food losses and waste throughout the system can help to maintain or improve consumption levels and at the same time alleviate pressures on production systems. The costs and benefits of a sustainable system must be reflected in decisions made by producers and consumers of food, as well as those who help shape decisions (FAO, 2012a).

Attempts to improve the sustainability of food systems face a number of challenges, such as market and non-market constraints to more diversified production and to higher levels of productivity, particularly for smallholders; unequal access to resources for women, the poor and other economically and socially marginalized groups; and increasing demands on natural resources, such as competition for water between agriculture and human settlements. In the context of weak governance, power asymmetries and the lack of clear and enforced property rights, production and consumption patterns are likely to be unsustainable. When combined with continuing inequities, the situation can have devastating consequences for nutrition, affecting both availability and accessibility of food, particularly for the poor.

Dietary diversity and nutrition

Healthy diets[5] contain a balanced and adequate combination of macronutrients (carbohydrates, fats and protein) and essential micronutrients (vitamins and minerals). Some questions remain controversial, such as whether animal-source foods are an essential part of the diet and whether all people, especially young children, can acquire adequate nutrients from food without

[5] We recognize that what constitutes a healthy diet is a matter of great debate and are therefore careful not to suggest what foods consumers should and should not consume. We do, however, report on efforts made to change consumption patterns based on others' judgements of what foods are more or less nutritious.

BOX 2
The importance of animal-source foods in diets

Animal foods are recognized as having high energy density and as good sources of high-quality protein; readily available iron and zinc; vitamins B_6, B_{12} and B_2; and, in liver, vitamin A. They enhance the absorption of iron and zinc from plant-based foods (Gibson, 2011). Evidence from the Nutrition Collaborative Research Support Programme (NCRSP) for Egypt, Kenya and Mexico indicated strong associations between the intake of foods from animal sources and better physical and cognitive development in children (Allen *et al.*, 1992; Neuman, Bwibo and Sigman, 1992; Kirksey *et al.*, 1992).

Increasing access to affordable animal-source foods could significantly improve nutritional status and health for many poor people, especially children. However, excessive consumption of livestock products is associated with increased risk of overweight and obesity, heart disease and other non-communicable diseases (WHO and FAO, 2003). Furthermore, the rapid growth of the livestock sector means that competition for land and other productive resources puts upward pressure on prices for staple grains as well as negative pressures on the natural resource base, potentially reducing food security in the longer term. Policy-makers need to take into consideration the trade-offs inherent when designing policies and interventions to promote animal-source foods.

Fish is also an important source of many nutrients, including protein of high quality, retinol, vitamins D and E, iodine and selenium. Evidence increasingly links the consumption of fish to enhanced brain development and learning in children, improved vision and eye health, and protection from cardiovascular disease and some cancers. The fats and fatty acids from fish are highly beneficial and difficult to obtain from other food sources. Evidence from Zambia documented that children whose main staple food is cassava and whose diets regularly include fish and other foods containing high-quality protein had a significantly lower prevalence of stunting than those whose diets did not (FAO, 2000).

supplementation (see Box 2 for a discussion of animal-source foods and diets). Nutrition guidelines generally maintain that diverse diets that combine a variety of cereals, legumes, vegetables, fruits and animal-source foods will provide adequate nutrition for most people to meet energy and nutrient requirements, although supplements may be needed for certain populations.

Nutritionists consider dietary diversity, or dietary variety – defined as the number of different foods or food groups consumed over a given reference period – as a key indicator of a high-quality diet (Ruel, 2003).[6] Evidence indicates that dietary diversity is strongly and positively associated with child nutritional status and growth, even after socio-economic factors have been controlled for (Arimond and Ruel, 2004; Arimond *et al.*, 2010).

Knowledge and information gaps

A significant body of direct and indirect evidence exists about the causal and synergistic links between food, agriculture and nutrition. The available knowledge, much of which is covered in this report, supports the proposition that the food and agriculture sector can play a central role in reducing malnutrition and that decisive policy action in this sector can improve nutritional outcomes, especially when accompanied by complementary interventions in education, health and sanitation, and social protection. Food system interventions can raise producers' incomes; improve the availability, affordability, acceptability and quality of food; and help

[6] Kennedy (2004) makes the point that while dietary diversity is generally beneficial, adding foods that are high in fats (energy) will not help to reduce overweight and obesity, so the nature of the diversity also needs to be taken into account. Experts differ on how to categorize foods into different groups, so "counting the diversity" of the diet is a complex task (Arimond *et al.*, 2010).

people make better food choices (Pinstrup-Andersen and Watson, 2011; Thompson and Amoroso, 2011; Fan and Pandya-Lorch, 2012).

Knowledge about many of the issues covered in this report remains incomplete, however. Many countries lack basic data and indicators for evaluating and monitoring the nutrition landscape. Agricultural interventions are difficult to evaluate[7] and many questions remain about the effectiveness of home gardens, the role of gender, agronomic fortification, technological innovations, biodiversity and the potential of local foods in the nutrition transition. Research on supply chain interventions and their impact on nutrition is scarce, but improved efficiency along the chain, reducing waste and losses, and raising the nutritional content of foods are among the least contentious issues in the food system and nutrition debate. The roles of trade, investment and market structure in nutritional outcomes remain contentious. Knowledge gaps also exist with regard to consumer choice and nutritional outcomes, and concepts such as "dietary diversity" and "healthy diets" remain fuzzy and difficult to measure objectively. Further research is needed on nutrition education and behaviour change, the link between food system policies and nutrition, and the nexus between the food industry, healthy diets and consumers. Finally, many questions remain about how food systems can contribute to better nutritional outcomes while also adhering to sustainable production and consumption patterns.

Structure of the report

Chapter 2 frames the debate by reviewing trends in malnutrition and illustrating how the transformation of food systems worldwide has been accompanied by dramatic changes in nutritional status. This implies that the nature of food system interventions to address malnutrition will vary according to the level of agricultural and economic development of a country and the nature of the malnutrition burden it faces. In all cases, however, making the food system more nutrition-sensitive can improve nutritional outcomes.

Chapter 3 looks at opportunities to enhance nutrition in agricultural production from inputs up to the farm gate. These include making general agricultural policies and institutions more nutrition-sensitive and employing nutrition-specific interventions to enhance the nutritional quality of staple crops, diversify production and improve farm management in ways that promote more nutritious and sustainable food systems.

Chapter 4 turns to nutrition-sensitive interventions in the supply chain from the farm gate to the retailer, through storage, processing and distribution. Food supply chains are evolving rapidly in all countries, and these changes have implications for the availability and affordability of diverse, nutritious foods for consumers in different areas and at different income levels. Specific interventions to enhance efficiency, reduce nutrient losses and waste and improve the nutritional content of foods can improve nutritional outcomes by making food more available, accessible, diverse and nutritious.

Chapter 5 focuses on interventions in the food system aimed at changing consumer behaviour. While these challenges relate more to education and behaviour change, they still involve improving the nutritional performance of the food system.

Chapter 6 provides an overview of global governance of the food system for better nutritional outcomes.

[7] The recent review by Masset *et al.* (2011) finds that a range of methodological and statistical reasons account for the sparse body of evidence by which to evaluate agricultural interventions.

2. Malnutrition and changing food systems

The multiple burdens of malnutrition – undernourishment and undernutrition, micronutrient deficiencies, and overweight and obesity – impose high and, in some cases, rising economic and social costs in countries at all income levels. Different types of malnutrition may coexist within the same country, household or individual, and their prevalence is changing rapidly along with changes in food systems. The often confusing terminology used to describe malnutrition is it itself a reflection of the complex, multidimensional, dynamic nature of the problem and the policy challenges associated with it.

Malnutrition concepts, trends and costs

Malnutrition is an abnormal physiological condition caused by inadequate, unbalanced or excessive consumption of the macronutrients that provide dietary energy (carbohydrates, protein and fats) and the micronutrients (vitamins and minerals) that are essential for physical and cognitive growth and development (FAO, 2011c). Good nutrition both depends on and contributes to good health.

Undernourishment and undernutrition

Undernourishment refers to food *intake* that is insufficient to meet dietary energy requirements for an active and healthy life. Undernourishment, or hunger, is estimated by FAO as the prevalence and number of people whose food intake is insufficient to meet their requirements on a continuous basis; dietary energy supply is used as a proxy for food intake. Since 1990–92, the estimated number of undernourished people in developing countries has declined from 980 million to 852 million and the prevalence of undernourishment has declined from 23 percent to 15 percent (FAO, IFAD and WFP, 2012).

Undernutrition is the *outcome* of insufficient food intake and repeated infections (UNSCN, 2010). Undernutrition or underweight in adults is measured by the body mass index (BMI), with individuals with a BMI of 18.5 or less considered to be underweight.[8]

Measures of undernutrition are more widely available for children: underweight (being too thin for one's age), wasting (being too thin for one's height) and stunting (being too short for one's age). This report uses stunting in children under the age of five as the primary indicator of undernutrition because stunting captures the effects of long-term deprivation and disease and is a powerful predictor of the life-long burden of undernutrition (Victora *et al.*, 2008).

Stunting is caused by long-term inadequate dietary intake and continuing bouts of infection and disease, often beginning with maternal malnutrition, which leads to poor foetal growth, low birth weight and poor growth. Stunting causes permanent impairment to cognitive and physical development that can lower educational attainment and reduce adult income. Between 1990 and 2011, the prevalence of stunting in developing countries declined by an estimated 16.6 percentage points, from 44.6 percent to 28 percent. There are 160 million stunted children in developing countries today, compared with 248 million in 1990 (UNICEF, WHO and The World Bank, 2012). Country-level malnutrition data mask considerable socio-economic or regional differences within countries. Although data are limited, a stark division between rural and urban areas in the burden of undernutrition is apparent in many countries (Box 3).

[8] The BMI equals the body weight in kilograms divided by height in metres squared (kg/m^2) and is commonly measured in adults to assess underweight, overweight and obesity. The international references are as follows: underweight = BMI $<$ 18.5; overweight = BMI $\geq$ 25; obese = BMI $\geq$ 30. Obesity is thus a subset of the overweight category.

BOX 3
The urban–rural malnutrition divide

Available cross-country evidence on child nutritional status consistently shows that, on average, children in urban areas are better nourished than children in rural areas (Smith, Ruel and Ndiaye, 2005; Van de Poel, O'Donnell and Van Doorslaer, 2007). The most recent data compiled by UNICEF (2013) shows that in 82 out of 95 developing countries for which data are available the prevalence of child underweight is higher in rural areas than in urban areas.

Evidence from India indicates that the rural–urban divide may also hold for adults. Guha-Khasnobis and James (2010) found a prevalence of adult underweight of around 23 percent in the slum areas of eight Indian cities, while the prevalence in rural areas in the same states was close to 40 percent. Headey, Chiu and Kadiyala (2011) argue that the combination of laborious farm employment and weaker access to education and health services jointly contribute to rural adult nutrition indicators being substantially worse than those of urban slum populations.

The socio-economic determinants of child nutritional status, such as maternal education and status within the family, are generally consistent between urban and rural areas, but the levels of these determinants often differ markedly between urban and rural areas. Urban mothers have approximately twice as much education and considerably higher decision-making power than their rural counterparts (Garrett and Ruel, 1999; Menon, Ruel and Morris, 2000).

Other evidence supporting the advantage of urban children over their rural counterparts is provided by country-level analyses. They show that urban children tend to have better access to health services, which in turn is reflected by higher immunization rates (Ruel *et al.*, 1998). Urban households are also more likely to have access to water and sanitation facilities, although they may come at high cost, especially for the poor (World Resources Institute, 1996). Finally, except for breastfeeding practices, which are more likely to be optimal among rural mothers, children's diets in urban areas are generally more diverse and more likely to include nutrient-rich foods such as meat, dairy products and fresh fruits and vegetables (Ruel, 2000; Arimond and Ruel, 2002). Examples from IFPRI's analysis of 11 demographic and health surveys show the consistently higher intake of milk and meat products by toddlers in urban areas compared with rural areas (Arimond and Ruel, 2004).

Thus, the lower prevalence of undernutrition among children in urban areas appears to be the result of the cumulative effect of a series of more favourable socio-economic conditions, which in turn lead to a healthier environment and better feeding and caring practices for children.

Micronutrient deficiencies

Micronutrient malnutrition is defined as being deficient in one or more vitamins and minerals of importance for human health. It is an *outcome* of inappropriate dietary composition and disease. It is technically a form of undernutrition (UNSCN, 2010), but is often referred to separately because it can coexist with adequate or excessive consumption of macronutrients and carries health consequences that are distinct from those associated with stunting.

Several micronutrients have been identified as being important for human health, but most of these are not widely measured. Three of the most commonly measured micronutrient deficiencies and related disorders refer to vitamin A, anaemia (related to iron) and iodine (Figure 2 and Annex table). Other micronutrients, such as zinc, selenium and vitamin B_{12}, are also important for health, but comprehensive data do not exist to provide global estimates of deficiencies in these micronutrients. This report also tends to report micronutrient deficiencies among children, again because data across countries are more consistently available for children than for adults.

Deficiency in vitamin A impairs normal functioning of the visual system and maintenance of cell function for growth, red blood cell production, immunity and reproduction (WHO, 2009). Vitamin A deficiency is the leading cause of blindness in children. In 2007, 163 million children under five in developing countries were estimated to be vitamin A deficient, with a prevalence of about 31 percent, down from approximately 36 percent in 1990 (UNSCN, 2010).[9]

Iron is important for red blood cell production. A deficiency in iron intake leads to anaemia (other factors also contribute to anaemia, but iron deficiency is the main cause). Iron-deficiency anaemia negatively affects the cognitive development of children, pregnancy outcomes, maternal mortality and the work capacity of adults. Estimates indicate modest progress overall in reducing iron-deficiency anaemia among children under five and pregnant and non-pregnant women (UNSCN, 2010).

Iodine deficiency impairs the mental function of 18 million children born each year. Overall, iodine deficiency – as measured by both total goitre rate and low urinary iodine – is falling. Estimates indicate that goitre prevalence (indicative of an extended period of deprivation, assessed in adults and/or children) in developing countries fell from around 16 percent to 13 percent between 1995–2000 and 2001–07 (regional averages shown for only two time periods in Figure 2 due to data limitations). Low urinary iodine (indicative of a current iodine deficiency) fell from around 37 percent to 33 percent (UNSCN, 2010).[10]

Despite considerable variation at country level (see Annex table), a number of regional and subregional trends and patterns in stunting and micronutrient deficiencies are discernible, as shown in Figure 2 and the Annex table.[11] In general, sub-Saharan Africa and Southern Asia have high levels of stunting and micronutrient deficiencies, with relatively modest improvements over the last two decades. Prevalence rates for stunting and micronutrient deficiencies are relatively low in Latin America and the Caribbean. In terms of numbers, most of the severely affected population lives in Asia, but with wide subregional variation.

Overweight and obesity

Overweight and obesity, defined as abnormal or excessive fat accumulation that may impair health (WHO, 2013a), are most commonly measured using BMI (see footnote 8 and Box 4). A high body mass index is recognized as increasing the likelihood of incurring various non-communicable diseases and health problems, including cardiovascular disease, diabetes, various cancers and osteoarthritis (WHO, 2011a). The health risks associated with overweight and obesity increase with the degree of excess body fat.

The global prevalence of combined overweight and obesity has risen in all regions, with prevalence among adults increasing from 24 percent to 34 percent between 1980 and 2008. The prevalence of obesity has increased even faster, doubling from 6 percent to 12 percent. (Figure 3) (Stevens *et al.*, 2012).

The prevalence of overweight and obesity is increasing in nearly all countries, even in low-income countries where it coexists with high rates of undernutrition and micronutrient deficiencies. Stevens *et al.* (2012) found that, in 2008, Central and South America, North Africa and the Middle East, Northern America and Southern Africa were the subregions with the highest prevalence of obesity (ranging from 27 percent to 31 percent).

Social and economic costs of malnutrition

The social and economic costs of malnutrition can be quantified in different ways, although any methodology has limitations. Disability-adjusted life years (DALYs) measure the social burden of disease, or the health gap

[9] The UNSCN (2010) estimates of the prevalence of vitamin A, iodine and anaemia deficiencies at the world, developing region and regional levels presented in Figure 2 are slightly different from those presented in the Annex table. The latter are calculated using weighted averages of the country prevalences reported in the Micronutrient Initiative (2009) report.

[10] Both sets of estimates are based on multivariate models applied to all countries for those time periods. The estimates are not very different from those obtained by simply averaging over the available surveys (UNSCN, 2010).

[11] Regional groupings follow the M49 UN classification. For more details, see Statistical annex.

FIGURE 2
Prevalence of stunting, anaemia and micronutrient deficiencies among children,* by developing region

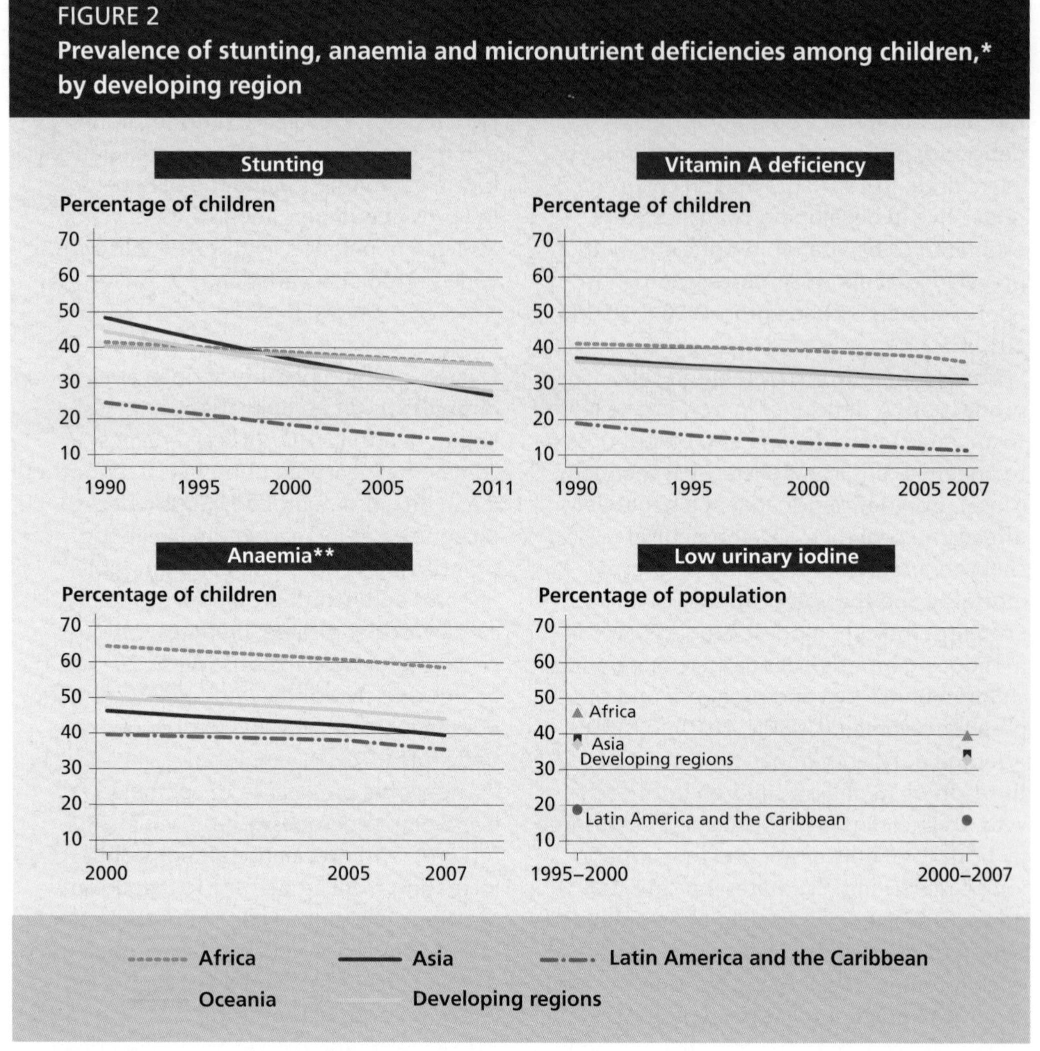

Notes: *Data for stunting, vitamin A deficiency and anaemia data refer to children under five years of age; data for low urinary iodine refer to the entire population.
**Anaemia is caused by several conditions, including iron deficiency.
Sources: Authors' compilation using data on stunting from UNICEF, WHO and The World Bank, 2012 (see also the Annex table of this report), and data on vitamin A deficiency, anaemia and low urinary iodine from UNSCN, 2010.

between current health status and an ideal situation where everyone lives into old age, free of disease and disability (WHO, 2008a). One DALY represents the loss of the equivalent of one full year of "healthy" life.

DALYs are used in a number of ways in making health policy decisions, including identifying national disease control priorities and allocating time for health practitioners and resources across health interventions and R&D (World Bank, 2006b). Because the DALY framework takes into account the interrelationships between nutrition, health and well-being (Stein *et al.*, 2005), it can also be used in economic analyses and assessments of the cost-effectiveness of health and nutrition interventions to assess the relative progress of health policies across countries (Robberstadt, 2005; Suárez, 2011).

The most recent work on the global burden of disease shows that child and maternal malnutrition still imposes by far the largest nutrition-related health burden globally, with more than 166 million DALYs lost per year in 2010 compared with 94 million DALYs lost due to adult overweight and obesity (Table 1). Worldwide, DALYs attributed to high BMI (overweight and obesity) and related risk factors, such as diabetes and high blood pressure, have increased dramatically, while those attributed to child and maternal malnutrition have decreased. However, in most of sub-Saharan Africa, child underweight remains

BOX 4
Limitations of using the body mass index in measuring excessive body fat

Body mass index (BMI) is a convenient and widely available measure of underweight, overweight and obesity. It is a proxy measure of excessive body fat. BMI does not distinguish between weight from fatty tissue and that from muscle tissue; nor does it indicate how an individual's body mass is distributed. People who carry a disproportionate amount of weight around their abdomen are at a higher risk of various health problems; waist circumference can therefore be a useful measure to gain additional insight, but it is measured less often and less easily than BMI (National Obesity Observatory, 2009).

BMI classifications were established based on risks of type 2 diabetes and cardiovascular disease, but populations and individuals vary in terms of how BMI relates to both body fat composition and the prevalence of disease (WHO, 2000).

The limitations of the international BMI classifications are particularly evident among Asian populations. For example, in 2002 an expert group, convened by the World Health Organization (WHO), found that the Asian populations considered have a higher percentage of body fat as well as higher incidence of diabetes and cardiovascular disease at lower BMIs than do Caucasians (controlling for age and sex). However, the experts also found differences in the appropriate BMI cut-off points among the Asian populations themselves. The expert group decided to maintain the existing international standard classifications, but also recommended the development of an additional classification system for Asian populations that uses lower cut-offs and encouraged the use of country-specific cut-offs and the waist circumference measure (Nishida, 2004).

FIGURE 3
Prevalence of overweight and obesity among adults, by region

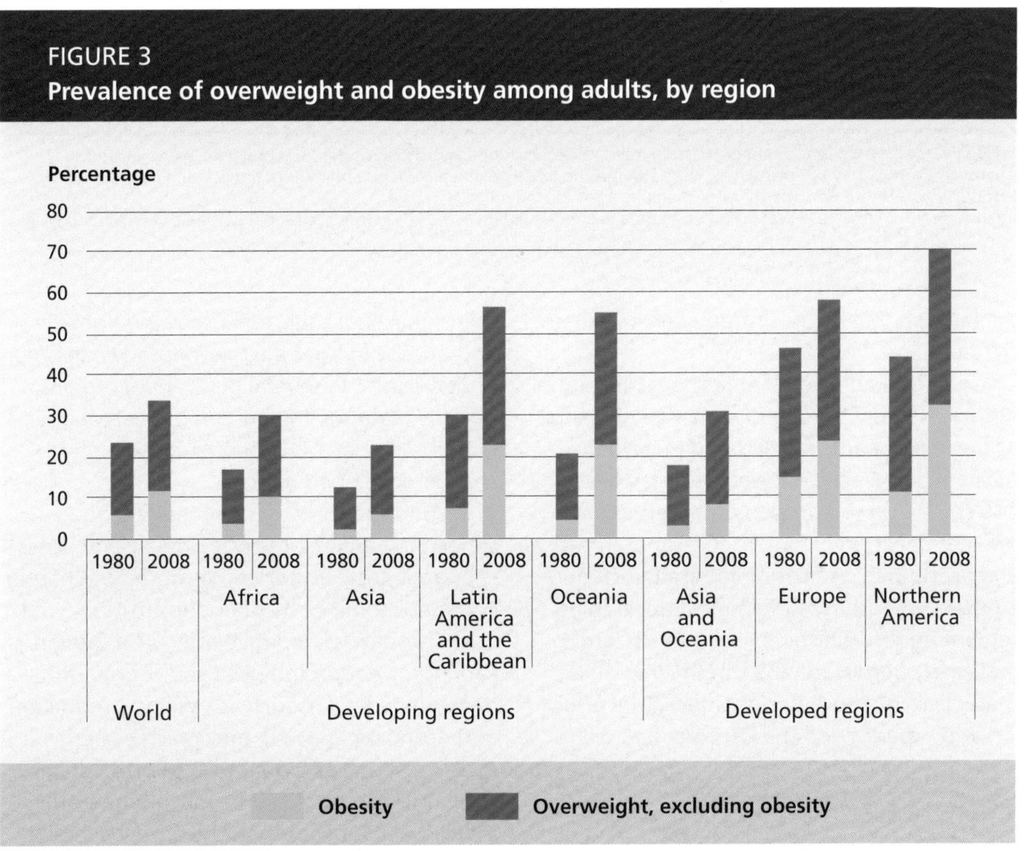

Sources: Authors' calculations using data presented in Finucane *et al.*, 2011 and Stevens *et al.*, 2012.

TABLE 1
Disability-adjusted life years in 1990 and 2010, by malnutrition-related risk factor, population group and region

REGION	CHILD AND MATERNAL MALNUTRITION		UNDERWEIGHT				OVERWEIGHT AND OBESITY			
	Total DALYs *(Thousands)*		Total DALYs *(Thousands)*		DALYS per 1 000 population *(Number)*		Total DALYs *(Thousands)*		DALYs per 1 000 population *(Number)*	
	1990	2010	1990	2010	1990	2010	1990	2010	1990	2010
World	**339 951**	**166 147**	**197 774**	**77 346**	**313**	**121**	**51 613**	**93 840**	**20**	**25**
Developed regions	**2 243**	**1 731**	**160**	**51**	**2**	**1**	**29 956**	**37 959**	**41**	**44**
Developing regions	**337 708**	**164 416**	**197 614**	**77 294**	**356**	**135**	**21 657**	**55 882**	**12**	**19**
Africa	**121 492**	**78 017**	**76 983**	**43 990**	**694**	**278**	**3 571**	**9 605**	**15**	**24**
Eastern Africa	42 123	21 485	27 702	11 148	779	205	353	1 231	5	11
Middle Africa	18 445	17 870	12 402	11 152	890	488	157	572	6	13
Northern Africa	10 839	4 740	4 860	1 612	216	68	2 030	4 773	36	47
Southern Africa	2 680	1 814	930	382	155	63	620	1 442	36	51
Western Africa	47 405	32 108	31 089	19 696	947	383	412	1 588	6	14
Asia	**197 888**	**80 070**	**115 049**	**32 210**	**297**	**90**	**12 955**	**34 551**	**9**	**16**
Central Asia	3 182	1 264	967	169	133	27	953	1 709	43	57
Eastern Asia	21 498	4 645	6 715	347	53	4	5 427	13 331	9	14
Southern Asia	138 946	60 582	89 609	27 325	514	150	2 953	9 281	6	11
South-Eastern Asia	27 971	9 736	15 490	3 318	270	61	1 045	5 032	5	16
Western Asia	6 291	3 843	2 269	1 051	104	41	2 577	5 198	42	45
Latin America and the Caribbean	**17 821**	**6 043**	**5 292**	**979**	**94**	**18**	**5 062**	**11 449**	**26**	**36**
Caribbean	2 559	1 073	849	252	204	67	401	854	25	38
Central America	5 437	1 491	2 124	366	133	22	1 228	3 309	28	42
South America	9 826	3 479	2 319	361	64	11	3 433	7 286	25	34
Oceania	**507**	**286**	**290**	**115**	**302**	**87**	**69**	**276**	**30**	**67**

Notes: DALY (disability-adjusted life year) estimates for child and maternal malnutrition include factors such as child underweight, iron deficiency, vitamin A deficiency, zinc deficiency and suboptimal breastfeeding. They also include maternal haemorrhage and maternal sepsis and iron-deficiency anaemia among women. Estimates for overweight and obesity refer to adults aged 25 and older.
Source: Compiled by the Institute for Health Metrics and Evaluation using data presented in Lim *et al.*, 2012 from the Global Burden of Disease Study 2010.

the leading risk factor underlying the disease burden (Lim *et al.*, 2012).

Population-adjusted DALYs show substantial decreases in the burden of underweight, one of the components of child and maternal malnutrition (Table 1).[12] Nevertheless, they also show that the burden of underweight remains particularly high in sub-Saharan Africa and in Southern Asia. Population-adjusted DALYs further show that in most developing regions underweight imposes a much larger cost than overweight and obesity (for their respective reference populations). Conversely, in Latin America and the Caribbean as well as in some Asian subregions, overweight and obesity impose a larger burden than underweight. In several developing regions, notably Oceania, the burden of overweight and obesity per 1 000 population is higher than in developed regions.

Beyond the social costs of malnutrition reflected in DALYs, malnutrition also imposes economic costs on society. As noted in Chapter 1, the economic costs of undernutrition, which arise through its negative effects on human capital formation (physical and cognitive development), productivity, poverty reduction and economic growth, may reach as high as 2–3 percent of global GDP (World Bank, 2006a). These costs can be much higher in individual countries than the global average implies. For example, one study estimated

[12] Population refers to the particular population group, i.e. children under five for underweight and adults for overweight and obesity.

the total cost of underweight for five Central American countries and the Dominican Republic at US$6.7 billion, ranging from 1.7 percent to 11.4 percent of GDP (Martínez and Fernández, 2008). Around 90 percent of the cost was accounted for by productivity losses due to higher mortality and lower educational attainment.

The economic costs of undernutrition are cumulative through an inter-generational life cycle of deprivation. An estimated 15.5 percent of babies are born each year with low birth weight (UNSCN, 2010). Low birth weight, childhood undernutrition, exposure to poor sanitary conditions and inadequate health care are reflected in poor physical growth and mental development, resulting in lower adult productivity.[13] In addition, the "developmental origins of adult disease" hypothesis (also known as the Barker hypothesis) posits that low birth weight has lasting negative health effects, such as being at greater risk of overweight, diabetes and coronary heart disease in adulthood (de Boo and Harding, 2006). More insidiously, stunted girls grow up to be stunted mothers, and maternal stunting is one of the strongest predictors for giving birth to a low-birth-weight infant. Maternal and child malnutrition thus perpetuate the cycle of poverty.

Micronutrient deficiencies, as distinct from undernutrition, also impose significant costs on society. The median total economic loss due to physical and cognitive impairment resulting from anaemia was estimated at 4 percent of GDP for ten developing countries, ranging from 2 percent in Honduras to 8 percent in Bangladesh (Horton and Ross, 2003). This study also suggested that while the productivity losses associated with anaemia are higher for individuals who must perform heavy manual work (17 percent), they are also serious for those doing light manual work (5 percent) and cognitive tasks (4 percent). Further evidence shows that treating anaemia can increase productivity even for people whose work is not physically demanding (Schaetzel and Sankar, 2002).

Vitamin and mineral deficiencies have been estimated to represent an annual loss of between 0.2 and 0.4 percent of GDP in China; this represents a loss of US$2.5–5.0 billion (World Bank, 2006a). Ma *et al.* (2007) found that actions to solve iron and zinc deficiencies in China would cost less than 0.3 percent of GDP, but failure to take action could result in a loss of 2–3 percent of GDP. For India, Stein and Qaim (2007) estimated that the combined economic cost of iron-deficiency anaemia, zinc deficiency, vitamin A deficiency and iodine deficiency amounts to around 2.5 percent of GDP.

Overweight and obesity also impose economic costs on society directly through increased health care spending and indirectly through reduced economic productivity. Most of the losses occur in high-income countries. A recent study by Bloom *et al.* (2011) estimates a cumulative output loss due to non-communicable diseases, for which overweight and obesity are key risk factors, of US$47 trillion over the next two decades; assuming a 5 percent rate of inflation, this would amount to around US$1.4 trillion, or 2 percent of global GDP in 2010.

A meta-analysis of 32 studies from 1990 to 2009 compared estimates of the direct costs of health care spending related to overweight and obesity in several high-income countries as well as in Brazil and China. Estimates of the direct costs for adults ranged from 0.7 percent to 9.1 percent of the individual countries' total health care expenditures. The cost of health care for overweight and obese people is around 30 percent higher than for other people (Withrow and Alter, 2010). In the United States of America, around 10 percent of total health care spending is obesity-related (Finkelstein *et al.*, 2009).

Total costs (direct and indirect costs) are, of course, higher. Total costs arising from overweight and obesity in the United Kingdom were estimated at £20 billion in 2007 (Government Office for Science, 2012). The indirect costs of overweight and obesity among adults in China were estimated at around US$43.5 billion (3.6 percent of GNP) in 2000, compared with direct costs of around US$5.9 billion (0.5 percent of GNP) (Popkin *et al.*, 2006).

Multiple burdens of malnutrition

The burdens of malnutrition can overlap, as shown in Figure 4. It is common to describe a double or even triple burden of malnutrition (FAO, IFAD and WFP, 2012), yet

[13] Alderman and Behrman (2004) calculate that the economic benefits from preventing one child from being born with a low birth-weight are about US$580 (the present discounted value).

the three types of malnutrition considered here (designated as A = child stunting, B = child micronutrient deficiencies and C = adult obesity) occur in different combinations around the world. The figure also shows the very few countries in the world that have no significant malnutrition problems in these categories.

The first group (AB) includes countries where rates of child stunting and micronutrient deficiencies are classified by the World Health Organization (WHO) as moderate or severe. All countries where stunting is a public health concern also have prevalence rates for micronutrient deficiencies classified by WHO as moderate or severe. The second group (B) includes countries where stunting rates have declined but micronutrient deficiencies remain widespread. These countries illustrate that simply addressing the factors influencing stunting, including increasing the energy content of diets, is not sufficient to provide the necessary range of micronutrients.

The next three groups include countries where the prevalence of adult obesity exceeds the global median. The third (ABC) includes countries where stunting, micronutrient deficiencies and obesity occur simultaneously. The fourth (BC) includes countries where the prevalence of stunting has declined but micronutrient deficiencies remain and obesity is a significant problem. Countries in the fifth group (C) have reduced stunting and micronutrient deficiencies but have serious obesity problems. Only 14 countries in this sample, all of them high-income countries, have no malnutrition problems of public health significance according to the malnutrition types and thresholds defined here.[14]

Food system transformation and malnutrition

The variations in malnutrition shown in Figure 4 reflect the changes in diets and lifestyles, known as the nutrition transition, that occur with economic growth and transformation of the food system. This process, also commonly referred to as agricultural transformation or the food system revolution, is typically characterized by rising labour productivity in agriculture, declining shares of population in agriculture and increasing rates of urbanization. As the food system transforms, centralized food-processing facilities develop along with large-scale wholesale and logistics companies, supermarkets emerge in the retail sector and fast-food restaurants become widespread. The transformation thus affects the whole system, changing the ways food is produced, harvested, stored, traded, processed, distributed, sold and consumed (Reardon and Timmer, 2012).

Figure 5 presents a stylized depiction of this transformation. In subsistence farming, the food system is basically "closed" – producers essentially consume what they produce. With economic development, subsistence farming gives way to commercial agriculture in which producers and consumers are increasingly separated in space and time and their interactions are mediated via markets. In the later stages of the food system transformation, very little overlap exists between producers and consumers and the system "opens up", reaching beyond the local economy to tie together producers and consumers, who may even live in different countries. The introduction of new actors may lead to consolidation of certain stages (for example, when wholesalers affiliated with supermarket chains buy directly from the producers and bypass the previous multiplicity of rural traders), but with additional processing the actual number of actors in the system may increase.

The relationships in Figure 6 are striking. All countries with agricultural GDP per worker below US$1 000 have severe problems of stunting *and* micronutrient deficiencies (category AB as described above). A large share of the population in these countries is rural and earns a living from agriculture. In Burundi, for example, 90 percent of the economically active population are in agriculture, and for all countries in this category this share is 62 percent.

As labour productivity rises to US$1 000–4 499 per worker, stunting declines sharply but all countries continue to suffer from micronutrient deficiencies, either alone

[14] Most of these countries may have nutrition-related public health concerns, but at rates below the thresholds defined here.

FIGURE 4
The multiple burdens of malnutrition

Category A: Child stunting

Category B: Child micronutrient deficiencies

Africa: Angola, Benin, Botswana, Burkina Faso, Burundi, Cameroon, Central African Republic, Chad, Comoros, Congo, Democratic Republic of the Congo, Côte d'Ivoire, Djibouti, Equatorial Guinea, Eritrea, Ethiopia, Gabon, Gambia, Ghana, Guinea, Guinea-Bissau, Kenya, Lesotho, Liberia, Madagascar, Malawi, Mali, Mauritania, Mozambique, Namibia, Niger, Nigeria, Rwanda, Sao Tome and Principe, Senegal, Sierra Leone, Somalia, Sudan,* Togo, United Republic of Tanzania, Uganda, Zambia, Zimbabwe

Asia: Afghanistan, Bangladesh, Bhutan, Cambodia, India, Indonesia, Democratic People's Republic of Korea, Lao People's Democratic Republic, Maldives, Mongolia, Myanmar, Nepal, Pakistan, Papua New Guinea, Philippines, Tajikistan, Turkmenistan, Timor-Leste, Viet Nam, Yemen

Latin America and the Caribbean: Bolivia (Plurinational State of), Haiti, Honduras

Africa: Algeria, Morocco

Asia: Brunei Darussalam, China, Kyrgyzstan, Malaysia, Sri Lanka, Thailand, Uzbekistan

Europe: Estonia, Romania

Latin America and the Caribbean: Brazil, Colombia, Guyana, Paraguay, Peru

Africa: Egypt, Libya, South Africa, Swaziland

Asia: Armenia, Azerbaijan, Iraq, Syrian Arab Republic

Europe: Albania

Latin America and the Caribbean: Belize, Ecuador, El Salvador, Guatemala

Oceania: Nauru, Solomon Islands, Vanuatu

Africa: Tunisia

Asia: Georgia, Iran (Islamic Rep. of), Jordan, Kazakhstan, Kuwait, Lebanon, Oman, Saudi Arabia, Turkey, United Arab Emirates

Europe: Belarus, Bosnia and Herzegovina, Bulgaria, Croatia, Latvia, Lithuania, The former Yugoslav Republic of Macedonia, Montenegro, Poland, Republic of Moldova, Russian Federation, Serbia, Slovakia, Ukraine

Latin America and the Caribbean: Argentina, Chile, Costa Rica, Cuba, Dominica, Dominican Republic, Jamaica, Mexico, Panama, Suriname, Trinidad and Tobago, Uruguay, Venezuela (Bolivarian Rep. of)

Oceania: Samoa, Tuvalu

Asia: Cyprus, Israel

Europe: Andorra, Czech Republic, Germany, Hungary, Iceland, Ireland, Portugal, Luxembourg, Malta, Slovenia, Spain, United Kingdom

Northern America: Canada, United States of America

Oceania: Australia, New Zealand

Category C: Adult obesity

Africa: Mauritius

Asia: Japan, Republic of Korea, Singapore

Europe: Austria, Belgium, Denmark, Finland, France, Greece, Italy, Netherlands, Norway, Sweden, Switzerland

Category D: No malnutrition problem of public health significance

Malnutrition category:

- Stunting and micronutrient deficiencies (AB)
- Micronutrient deficiencies (B)
- Micronutrient deficiencies and obesity (BC)
- Stunting, micronutrient deficiencies and obesity (ABC)
- Obesity (C)
- No malnutrition problem (D)

Notes: Data for stunting among children are from UNICEF, WHO and The World Bank (2012). A country is designated as having a public health threat related to stunting if at least 20 percent of its children are stunted (WHO, 2013b); data on stunting are not available for some high-income countries and these countries are assumed to have a prevalence of stunting that is far lower than 20 percent. Data on anaemia and vitamin A deficiency among children are from Micronutrient Initiative (2009). Countries face micronutrient deficiency-related public health threats if 10 percent or more of their children are deficient in vitamin A (WHO, 2009) or if at least 20 percent of children suffer from anaemia (WHO, 2008b). Countries with a per capita GDP of at least US$15 000 are assumed to be free of vitamin A deficiency (Micronutrient Initiative, 2009). Data on obesity among adults are from WHO (2013c). Countries where 20 percent or more of the adult population are obese (equivalent to the global median prevalence for that indicator) are considered to be facing a public health threat related to obesity.
* Data for Sudan was collected prior to 2011 and refer therefore to Sudan and South Sudan.
Source: Croppenstedt *et al.*, 2013. See also Annex table.

FIGURE 5
The food system transformation

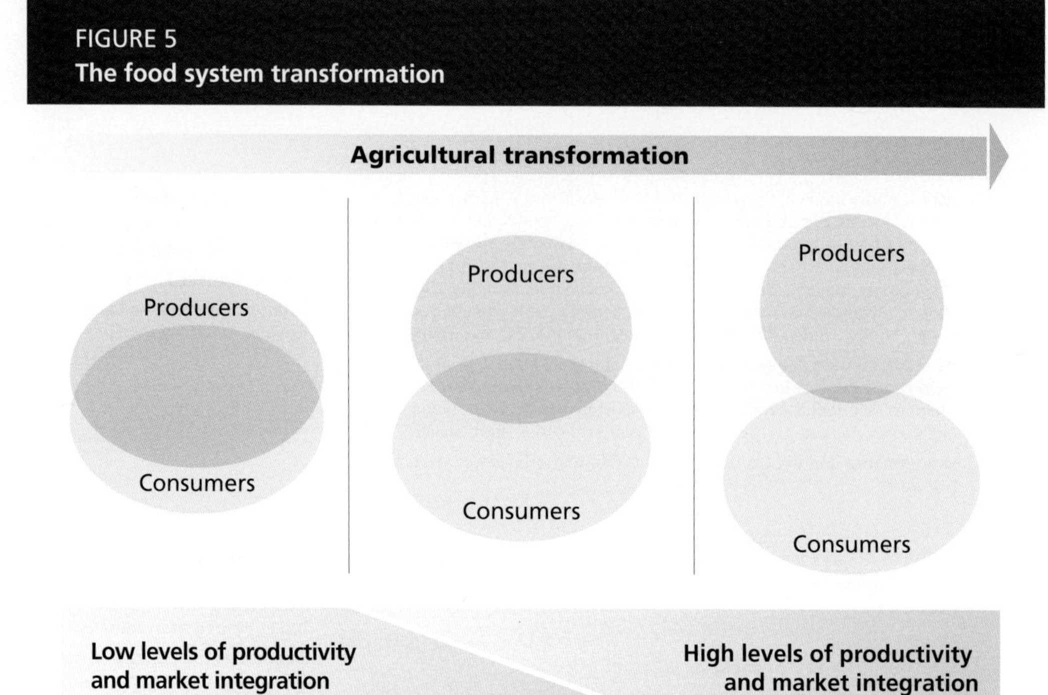

Source: FAO.

FIGURE 6
Share of countries in each malnutrition category, by level of agricultural productivity

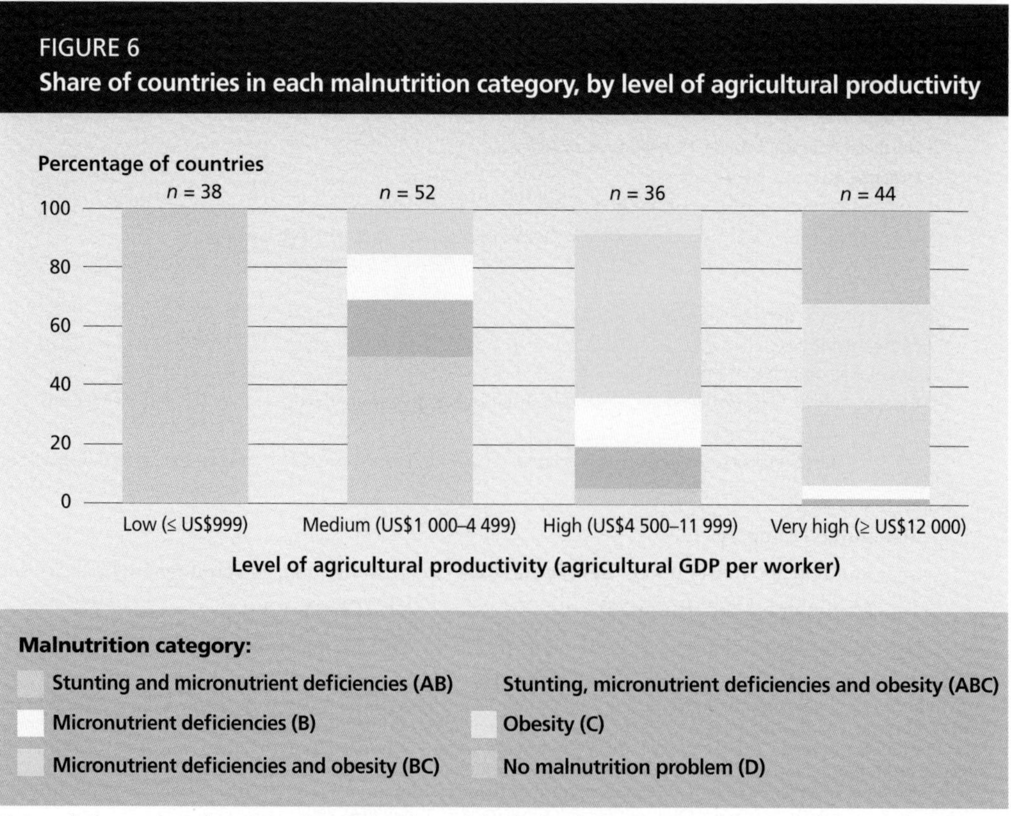

Notes: n is the number of countries characterized by each level of agricultural productivity. Agricultural productivity is derived by dividing agricultural GDP (in 2010 measured in current US dollars) by the population economically active in agriculture. Malnutrition categories are those illustrated in Figure 4.
Sources: Authors' calculations using agricultural GDP data from the United Nations (2012) and data on agricultural workers from FAO, 2013. Sources used to determine malnutrition categories are those used for Figure 4.

(category B) or in combination with stunting (AB), obesity (BC) or both (ABC). Already, at this medium level of agricultural labour productivity, obesity is a public health problem in more than one-third of all countries, always in combination with micronutrient deficiencies. Agriculture is still an important part of the economy in these countries, although the average share of the labour force in agriculture is lower, at 45 percent.

As labour productivity in agriculture rises above US$4 500, few countries continue to suffer from stunting, though most that do also add obesity to their woes (ABC). The majority of these relatively well-off countries suffer from micronutrient deficiencies and obesity (BC). Once agricultural labour productivity reaches very high levels per-worker, above US$12 000, a majority of countries manage to eliminate micronutrient deficiencies and a significant number manage to solve all three malnutrition problems. These countries typically have a very small share of the population in agriculture, are highly urbanized and have food systems that are globally integrated.

Figure 7 depicts this transition as it accompanies greater urbanization. The transformation of the malnutrition situation is remarkable and strikingly similar to that shown by growth in agricultural labour productivity: stunting falls and obesity rises almost in tandem. At the same time, micronutrient deficiencies fall very slowly as the rates of urbanization rise, and they remain remarkably prevalent even in higher-income, highly urbanized countries.

These changes in the food system, in agriculture and in levels of urbanization pose significant challenges. The nature of the malnutrition problem will itself transition, but problems of undernutrition, associated with deprivation, will continue to pose a major nutritional challenge, especially in low-income countries.

Dietary diversity in changing food systems

One of the key means of addressing micronutrient deficiencies – which seem to persist even with agricultural transformation, increased urbanization and higher incomes

FIGURE 7
Share of countries in each malnutrition category, by degree of urbanization

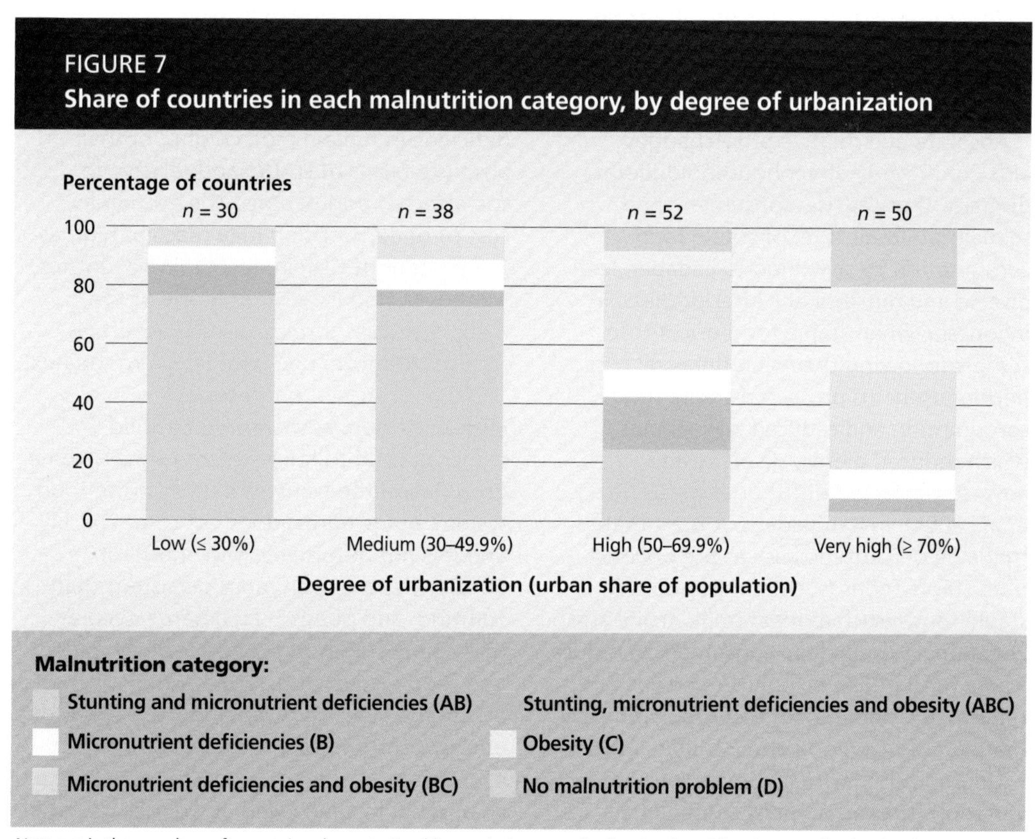

Notes: n is the number of countries characterized by each degree of urbanization. The degree of urbanization is the share of the urban population in the total population. Malnutrition categories are those illustrated in Figure 4.
Sources: Authors' calculations, using data for total and urban population from FAO, 2013. Sources used to determine malnutrition categories are those used for Figure 4.

– is through consumption of a high-quality, diverse diet. The relationship between dietary diversity and changes in food systems is complex. Dietary diversity is determined by relative prices, incomes and the tastes and preferences of individuals and households, all of which are affected by changes in food systems. Evidence at the global level strongly suggests that rising household incomes lead to greater variety in the diet. At higher incomes, an increasing share of the household's diet comes from animal products, vegetable oils and fruits and vegetables, that is, non-staples. Meat and dairy consumption increases strongly with income growth; fruit and vegetable consumption increases also but more slowly, and consumption of cereals and pulses declines (Regmi *et al.*, 2001).

Household surveys from Bangladesh, Egypt, Ghana, India, Kenya, Malawi, Mexico, Mozambique and the Philippines also find that dietary diversity is strongly associated with household consumption expenditure (Hoddinott and Yohannes, 2002). Evidence from Bangladesh shows that income growth leads to strong growth in expenditures on meat, fish, fruits and eggs but little change in expenditure on rice, a staple (Thorne-Lyman *et al.*, 2010).

Absolute and relative price changes also significantly affect household dietary diversity. If prices rise, consumers tend to maintain their level of staple food consumption by switching to cheaper, less-diverse and nutritionally inferior diets. In Indonesia, when staple food prices rose sharply following the Asian financial crisis, poor households protected staple food consumption and reduced non-staples, which reduced dietary diversity and adversely affected nutritional status (Block *et al.*, 2004). In Bangladesh, it is estimated that a 50 percent increase in the price of both staple foods (such as rice) and non-staple foods (such as meat, milk, fruits and vegetables) would lead consumers to reduce staple food intake by only 15 percent but reduce non-staple foods disproportionately more (Bouis, Eozenou and Rahman, 2011).

Households may react similarly to price variations that accompany seasonality; for example, a Save the Children pilot programme in the United Republic of Tanzania found that dietary diversity diminished during the lean season before harvest (Nugent, 2011). In such situations, social protection instruments are needed to avoid a deterioration in nutritional outcomes as well as to help households maintain assets, both human and physical, so as to prevent a short-term shock from turning into a long-term disaster.

Conclusions and key messages

The nature of the malnutrition burden facing the world is increasingly complex. Significant progress has been made in reducing food insecurity, undernourishment and undernutrition; however, prevalence rates remain high in some regions, most notably in sub-Saharan Africa and in Southern Asia. At the same time, micronutrient deficiencies remain stubbornly high and rates of overweight and obesity are rising rapidly in many regions, even in countries where undernutrition persists.

The social and economic costs of undernutrition, micronutrient deficiencies, and overweight and obesity are high. While costs associated with overweight and obesity are rising rapidly, those associated with undernutrition and micronutrient deficiencies remain much higher both in absolute terms of DALYs and relative to the affected populations. The economic cost of undernutrition may reach as high as 2–3 percent of GDP in developing countries. Moreover, undernutrition is one of the main pathways through which poverty is transmitted from one generation to the next.

Evidence shows that rates of undernutrition, as measured by child stunting, tend to fall with per capita income growth and the transformation of the food system, but progress does not come quickly and it is not automatic. Micronutrient deficiencies are even more persistent than stunting, and obesity can emerge even at fairly early stages of economic development and food system transformation.

Dietary diversity, given adequate levels of energy consumption, is a key determinant of nutritional outcomes but it is sensitive to changes in income levels and prices of staple and non-staple foods. In the face of a shock to food prices or incomes, households tend to maintain a minimum level of staple food consumption even if it means sacrificing more nutritious foods that are necessary to provide the vitamins and minerals needed for good health.

Food system transformation and the nutrition transition go hand in hand. To address the nutritional challenges in a given context it is first necessary to understand the nature of the food system and identify key entry points throughout the system. The next three chapters of this report look at the various stages of the food system to identify the major pathways through which food system interventions can improve nutritional outcomes.

Key messages

- Malnutrition in all its forms imposes unacceptably high costs on society in human and economic terms. Globally, the social burdens associated with undernutrition and micronutrient deficiencies are still much larger than those associated with overweight and obesity. Rural people in low- and middle-income countries bear by far the highest burden of malnutrition. Addressing undernutrition and micronutrient deficiencies must remain the highest priority of the global nutrition community, even as efforts are made to prevent or reverse the emergence of obesity.
- All forms of malnutrition share a common cause: inappropriate diets that provide inadequate, unbalanced or excessive macronutrients and micronutrients. The only sustainable means of addressing malnutrition is through the consumption of a high-quality, diverse diet that provides adequate but not excessive energy. Food systems determine the availability, affordability, diversity and quality of the food supply and thus play a major role in shaping healthy diets.
- Income growth, whether from agriculture or other sources, is closely associated with reductions in undernutrition, but income growth alone is not enough. It must be accompanied by specific actions aimed at improving dietary adequacy and quality if rapid progress is to be made in eradicating undernutrition and micronutrient deficiencies.
- Dietary diversity is a key determinant of nutritional outcomes, but the consumption of nutrient-dense foods is very sensitive to income and price shocks, especially for low-income consumers. Protecting the nutritional quality of diets – not just the adequacy of staple food consumption – should be a priority for policy-makers.
- The malnutrition burden in a country changes rapidly with the transformation of the food system. Policy-makers must therefore understand the specific nature of the malnutrition problem to design interventions throughout the food system. Up-to-date data and analysis are necessary to support decision-making.

3. Agricultural production for better nutrition[15]

Many opportunities exist to increase the contribution of agricultural production to improving nutrition. This chapter reviews strategies for enhancing the nutritional performance of agricultural production in three main areas: making food more available and accessible; making food more diverse and production more sustainable; and making food itself more nutritious.

Making food more available and accessible

The most fundamental way in which agricultural production contributes to nutrition is by making food more available and affordable through agricultural productivity growth. This strategy is particularly appropriate in settings where undernutrition and micronutrient deficiencies are the primary malnutrition concern. The foundation of the strategy rests on enhancing the productivity of the agriculture sector and providing an enabling environment for agricultural investment and growth (FAO, 2012c). The economic pathways through which productivity growth in agriculture makes food more available and affordable are through income growth, broader economic growth and poverty reduction, and lower real food prices.

Agricultural productivity growth and malnutrition

One of the key drivers of agricultural productivity growth is agricultural R&D. The introduction of higher-yielding varieties of rice, wheat and maize during the Green Revolution led to major improvements in nutrition through higher incomes and lower prices for staple foods (Alston, Norton and Pardey, 1995). It has been estimated that world food and feed prices would be 35–65 percent higher, average caloric availability 11–13 percent lower and the percentage of children malnourished in developing countries 6–8 percent higher had the Green Revolution not occurred (Evenson and Rosegrant, 2003).

Agricultural R&D for staple food productivity growth continues to be one of the most effective means of reducing hunger and food insecurity. Estimates from Madagascar show that a doubling of rice yields would reduce the share of households that are food-insecure by 38 percent, shorten the average hungry period by one-third, increase real unskilled wages in the lean season by 89 percent (due to both price and labour demand effects) and benefit all of the poor, including unskilled workers, consumers and net-selling rice farmers. Moreover, it would provide the biggest gains to the poorest through lower food prices and higher real wages for unskilled workers (Minten and Barrett, 2008).

Productivity growth allows farmers to produce more food with the same amount of resources, making the sector more economically efficient and environmentally sustainable. Farmers benefit directly: they earn higher incomes and can use the extra production to enhance their own household food consumption. In a second round of benefits, productivity growth enables farmers to hire additional workers and buy other goods and services, creating "multiplier effects" that can ripple throughout the economy, stimulating overall economic growth and reducing poverty (Hayami *et al.*, 1978; David and Otsuka, 1994).

Agricultural growth has been found to be much more effective than general economic growth at reducing poverty for the very poor. Growth in agriculture reduces 1 dollar-a-day headcount poverty more than three times faster than growth in non-agricultural sectors (Christiaensen, Demery and Kuhl, 2011). The

[15] This chapter is based in part on Miller and Welch (2012).

income and poverty effects of agricultural productivity growth are, of course, strongest in countries where agriculture is a large part of the economy and employs a large share of the labour force.

Several recent studies have established that sustained income growth, whether from agriculture or other sources, can have a sizeable effect on reducing malnutrition. For example, relatively strong, sustained per capita income growth of 2.5 percent per year for 20 years (a total of approximately 65 percent increase in income), would reduce the prevalence of underweight among children in developing countries by only 27 percent (Haddad *et al.*, 2003). Using regression analysis to adjust for several factors, Headey (2011) found that agricultural growth had a large effect in reducing stunting and underweight among children in the majority of the 89 surveys included in his sample. The amount of reduction resulting from growth in agriculture production and productivity depends greatly on a country's economic structure and the characteristics of malnutrition (Ecker, Breisinger and Pauw, 2011; Headey, 2011).

However, the relationship between agricultural and economic growth and improved nutrition is not automatic. India has experienced rapid agricultural and economic growth accompanied by improvements in most indicators of undernutrition among children, but the rate of progress has been far slower than that seen in other parts of the world and the prevalence of undernutrition remains among the highest in the world (Deaton and Drèze, 2009).

A closer look at available data describing periods of success or failure in reducing child malnutrition reveals a more nuanced picture. Agricultural productivity growth was associated with reductions in the prevalence of child malnutrition in most countries, including India, during the period of rapid adoption of Green Revolution technologies and up until the early 1990s. Since 1992, however, agricultural growth has not been associated with improved nutrition among children in many Indian states (Headey, 2011).

Various explanations have been offered for the persistence of high levels of undernutrition in India. These include economic inequality, gender inequality, poor hygiene, lack of access to clean water and other factors beyond the performance of the agriculture sector. However, the phenomenon remains largely unexplained and additional research is needed (Deaton and Drèze, 2009; Headey, 2011). The available evidence shows that agricultural and economic growth is effective in sustainably reducing malnutrition in low-income countries where many people depend on agriculture, but the impact is slow and may not be sufficient. Therefore, additional complementary ways to reduce malnutrition are necessary.

In addition to raising incomes and reducing poverty, agricultural productivity growth benefits consumers, both rural and urban. Through reducing the real price of food, it makes food more available and accessible, providing people with the opportunity to consume better diets. Lower real food prices enable consumers to fulfil their staple food requirements with a smaller share of their household budget, which means they can diversify their diets with other nutrient-dense foods such as meat, milk, fruits and vegetables.

Figure 6 (see page 22) shows the relationship between agricultural GDP-per-worker and the burden of malnutrition. It suggests that relatively high levels of agricultural productivity are needed before people diversify their diets sufficiently to satisfy their micronutrient needs. For young children, other mediating factors may inhibit the impact of income growth on nutrition, such as parental education, women's social status and access to health care and clean water.

Agricultural policy for better nutrition

Appropriate agricultural policies can influence agricultural productivity and nutritional outcomes, but such policies rarely have enhanced nutrition as a primary policy objective. Agricultural policies in many countries are quite complex and may influence nutrition in contradictory ways. Their impacts on nutrition may also vary according to the economic and nutritional context of the country. Agricultural policies that provide appropriate incentives and clear market signals that promote the sustainable intensification and diversification of production will improve nutrition more effectively.

Making food more available and accessible benefits people who are at risk of food insecurity and undernutrition; however, some have blamed agricultural policies in Organisation for Economic Co-operation and Development (OECD) countries for increasing overweight and obesity by making processed foods more widely available and cheaper than foods such as fruits and vegetables (Schäfer Elinder, 2005; Schoonover and Muller, 2006; Mozaffarian *et al.*, 2012). On the other hand, the Common Agricultural Policy in European countries actually raises consumer prices of sugar and dairy products relative to prices of fruits and vegetables and thus may have a small positive impact on the overall healthiness of European diets (Capacci *et al.*, 2012). Similarly, Alston, Sumner and Vosti (2006) found that agricultural subsidies in the United States of America have relatively small and mixed impacts on the prices of farm commodities, raising sugar prices and lowering maize prices, for example. They concluded that eliminating farm subsidies in the United States of America would have negligible consequences for overweight and obesity rates. Schmidhuber (2007) cautioned that whereas the Common Agricultural Policy served largely as a tax on consumers in the European Union (EU), it may have depressed prices and encouraged overconsumption in countries that imported food from the EU.

Hawkes *et al.* (2012) considered the impact of agricultural policies on diets throughout the world. They hypothesized that market liberalization since the 1980s has made food more readily available and affordable in many countries, but because both more nutritious and less nutritious foods have been affected, they concluded that this has had both positive and negative implications for the overall healthiness of diets. With rising incomes and increased affordability of a range of foods, factors such as convenience and responsiveness to nutrition education may be key variables in determining the effects of agricultural policies on nutrition.

In addition to the commodity support policies common in OECD countries, many developing countries subsidize agricultural inputs, mainly fertilizer and seeds, with a view to boosting smallholder crop production and achieving national food self-sufficiency. Levels of agricultural support in OECD and developing countries have converged since the 1980s, with the former falling significantly while the latter have risen (FAO, 2012c). Evidence from farm input subsidy programmes in India and Malawi indicates that they can significantly boost agricultural production and farmers' incomes, albeit at a high budgetary cost (HLPE, 2012), but the impact of such policies on nutrition has not been well studied. Input subsidies can be beneficial if targeted to specific groups, such as women, who are relatively more constrained in their access to commercial inputs (FAO, 2011b). As noted below, fertilizer subsidies may also have some nutritional public good attributes, with benefits to a wider population beyond the immediate beneficiaries. In general, the costs of input subsidies and their indirect effect on nutrition probably mean that other, more targeted, nutrition interventions would be more effective.

Gender and seasonal considerations

Efforts to boost agricultural productivity must also consider the impacts on time use – especially of women, who bear a greater responsibility for food preparation and child care (FAO, 2011b). Maternal and child nutrition are particularly vulnerable to the seasonal time demands placed on female agricultural workers. Disruptions to adequate maternal nutrition and good care and feeding practices during the critical "1 000 days" from conception through the first two years of life can cause lasting damage to women's health and life-long physical and cognitive impairment in children (Box 5). Understanding the nutritional consequences of the time constraints on rural women, investing in infrastructure and technology to alleviate these burdens and making specific nutrition-related interventions during critical periods in the agricultural calendar can help improve nutritional outcomes for women and children.

Agricultural interventions need to take into account the effect of seasonality on nutritional outcomes. Vaitla, Devereux and Swan (2009) note that much of the undernutrition in the world is due to the annual "hunger season". Particularly in areas dependent on rain-fed cultivation, the year-to-year availability of food is the key determinant of fluctuations in undernutrition

BOX 5
The first thousand days

Maternal and child undernutrition is the primary pathway through which poverty is transmitted from one generation to the next. About a quarter of all children under the age of five are stunted and about half suffer from one or more deficiencies in a key micronutrient. The critical window for adequate child growth and cognitive development is between conception and 24 months of age. Developmental damage that results from undernutrition during this period cannot be reversed or regained over time. For this reason, many national and international nutrition initiatives now focus on the first 1 000 days.

A recent series of articles in *The Lancet* in 2008 recommended a number of strategies for addressing undernutrition in mothers and young children, from which Horton *et al*. (2010) identified 13 highly cost-effective interventions. These interventions emphasized care and feeding practices, such as improved hygiene and de-worming, exclusive breastfeeding for infants during the first six months, and vitamin and mineral supplements. Food system interventions identified in this work were limited primarily to the provision of micronutrients through fortified foods.

Food fortification can certainly make an important contribution, but food systems can do even more to improve maternal and child nutrition during the crucial first 1 000 days. For example, while children should be exclusively breastfed for their first six months, after this time they need energy-dense, micronutrient-rich complementary foods, and older children gradually share what should be nutritious family diets. Food systems play an important role in providing, in a sustainable manner, diverse and nutritious food obtained from own production or from local markets. Nutrition education and counselling play a central role in promoting good prenatal and postnatal care and diets for the mother and child. This especially concerns the most appropriate types of complementary foods, as well as preparation, storage and feeding practices that help preserve or even increase the nutritional quality of the food (Hotz and Gibson, 2005).

Within the food system, gender roles are directly relevant for child and maternal malnutrition. Increasing women's control over resources and incomes has been shown to benefit their children's health, nutrition and education, as well as their own health and nutritional status (FAO, 2011b; World Bank, 2011). Agricultural production and food processing are the main sources of employment for women in most developing regions, yet women typically control fewer resources and earn lower incomes than men, so closing the gender gap in agriculture could produce significant nutritional gains for society, including during the first 1 000 days (FAO, 2011b).

Women in most countries also undertake most of the work related to child care, food preparation and other household responsibilities such as collecting fuel and water. Women thus face multiple trade-offs in the allocation of their time that directly impinge on their own and their children's health and nutritional status. As these trade-offs can be exacerbated by the seasonal nature of agricultural activities, attention should be paid to the effects that working conditions may have on a family's ability to care for its children. Policies, interventions and investment in labour-saving farming technologies and rural infrastructure, targeted safety nets, and services such as on-site child care can contribute significantly to health and nutritional outcomes for women, infants and young children.

and short-term deprivation (Kumar, 1987). In Malawi and the Niger, Cornia, Deotti and Sassi (2012) found that strong seasonal food price variations are a major determinant of child malnutrition; these fluctuations occur even in periods of relatively abundant harvests because of limited investment in storage at the community and household levels, limited credit availability and inadequate strategic food reserves.

Dietary energy requirements for agricultural households are higher during the harvest period, and food consumption increases if household food stores are adequate. In the Gambia, Kennedy and Bouis (1993) found that pregnant women were not able to compensate for higher energy expenditure during the season of peak agricultural labour demand. As a consequence, birth weights were below the international average for deliveries occurring after this period. During non-peak seasons, birth weights were close to international norms. The rainy season also coincides with increased incidence of disease, which further raises nutritional requirements. Heavy farm work coinciding with disease and reduced food availability are partly responsible for the difference in prevalence of malnutrition among rural and urban adults.

Making food more diverse

Sustained agricultural productivity growth, income growth and poverty reduction – whether from agriculture or other sources – can improve nutritional outcomes, but the mixed impacts of agricultural policies and the slow impacts of agricultural R&D on productivity growth suggest that there is room for improvement. Specific interventions aimed at diversifying what farmers produce and what food households have access to (e.g. through home gardens or raising small animals) can contribute to better nutrition.

Diversification at national scale

Agricultural policies, including R&D, can be used to make the food supply more diverse, although few countries have made diversification a specific policy objective. Some European governments have attempted to use agricultural policies to improve diets by reducing support for foods considered to be less healthy and investing more in other foods such as fruits and vegetables. In Finland, for example, the government implemented agricultural policy reform along with media and education campaigns to encourage the production and consumption of healthier foods. The reform included reducing subsidies for dairy products in favour of lean meats and promoting the production and consumption of berries (Mozaffarian *et al.*, 2012).

Agricultural R&D could be made more nutrition-sensitive by being more inclusive of small producers and focusing more resources on important non-staple foods and integrated production systems. Relatively little public agricultural R&D focuses on increasing the productivity of nutrient-dense foods such as fruits, vegetables, legumes and animal-source foods. Improved productivity would reduce the relative prices of these foods and could support dietary diversity. Post-harvest research could extend the limited seasonal availability and reduce the nutrient losses and food safety hazards associated with these highly perishable foods (see Chapter 4).

Diversifying home and small farm food production

Increasing micronutrient availability for poor households with limited access to land, in both urban and rural areas, is a particular challenge. Projects that support the diversification of home and smallholder production hold potential for improving consumption of a variety of foods and reducing micronutrient deficiencies. For example, in Kenya and the United Republic of Tanzania, a project aimed at promoting the production, marketing and consumption of traditional African vegetables among smallholders found that increasing crop diversity was associated with increased dietary diversity (Herforth, 2010).

The specific nature of these interventions depends on the type of agriculture practised and the type of constraints that households face in a given location. Such projects can range from small-scale home garden projects to more complex integrated farming projects (see Boxes 6 and 7).

Small-scale home gardens are promising interventions when micronutrient deficiencies are significant and fruit and vegetable consumption is low. Home gardening is already widely practised, can be effective on a small scale and is feasible in most locations, although water and labour constraints may pose challenges and should be carefully considered in project design.

A recent review found that most evaluations of home garden programmes were not designed to enable the assessment of impacts on nutritional status. Such studies did demonstrate increased consumption of fruits and vegetables, but the overall effect on nutrient consumption could not be assessed because they typically ignored substitution effects (Masset *et al.*, 2011).

Experience has also shown that home garden projects are more likely to be effective when accompanied by nutrition information and education and by a focus on roles traditionally held by women (such as child care and food preparation) as well as women's empowerment (World Bank, 2007a). Programmes in West Africa (Box 6) and Ethiopia (Box 7) illustrate the benefits that can accrue to such integrated action.

In some communities, micronutrient intakes can be enhanced more effectively by strengthening animal husbandry. For example, in Ethiopia, the important role of goats in the mixed farming systems of the high- and mid-altitude areas led to development of the FARM-Africa Dairy Goat Development Project (Ayele and Peacock, 2003). The project focused on increasing income and milk consumption by raising the productivity of local goats managed by women through a combination of improved management techniques and genetic improvements. The intervention led to an increase in the per capita availability of milk by 119 percent, energy from animal sources by 39 percent, protein by 39 percent and fat by 63 percent. Through impact analysis of data on those households within the project area, FARM-Africa demonstrated a considerable improvement in the nutritional status and family welfare of project participants (Ayele and Peacock, 2003).

Few of the home production interventions that target nutrition have been successfully scaled up. One exception is the Homestead Food Production (HFP) project, introduced in Bangladesh by Helen Keller International nearly two decades ago. This project initially focused on reducing vitamin A deficiency by promoting home gardens, but its scope has been widened to address iron and zinc deficiencies also by incorporating small-animal husbandry and nutrition education (Iannotti, Cunningham and Ruel, 2009). Implemented by non-governmental organization (NGO) partners and the Government of Bangladesh, HFP has expanded its reach into over one-half of the country's subdistricts and has been extended to other countries in Asia and sub-Saharan Africa.

BOX 6
Increasing dietary diversity through home gardens

Action Contre La Faim (ACF) developed an approach in West Africa based on home vegetable gardens aimed at promoting good nutrition at the household level by diversifying supply and increasing dietary diversity. This approach, called "Health & Nutrition Gardens" also aims at empowering women to sustain good nutrition in their families. Apart from facilitating access to inputs, training on crop production, and post-harvest conservation, ACF's approach also includes:

- evaluation of food consumption patterns;
- selection of micronutrient-rich vegetables to enrich deficient diets;
- research into recipes that seek to provide a balanced diet based on local foods;
- cooking demonstrations;
- awareness-raising and nutrition education to improve maternal and child-feeding practices.

The results have been positive. The supply of vegetables has increased by over 160 percent and vegetables are now available for nine months of the year, compared with five months before the programme. Dietary diversity at the household level has improved and consumption, especially of foods rich in vitamin A, has improved markedly. Participants' knowledge of the causes of malnutrition has also increased to 88 percent compared with 68 percent among non-participants.

The positive experience with these "Health & Nutrition Gardens" has led ACF to scale up the programme in West Africa, as well as in Asia, the Caucasus and Central and South America.

Source: Contributed by ACF International.

BOX 7
Improving child nutrition in small-scale pastoral food systems

Child malnutrition is severe among pastoral communities in the Somali region of Ethiopia, (Mason *et al*., 2010). A substantial proportion of the population's dietary intake and income is derived from livestock products. Save the Children's Milk Matters project aimed to improve the ways that animal husbandry and livestock production can benefit the nutritional status of local children.

In the first phase of the project, a participatory approach was used to identify which factors pastoralists considered the most important in affecting the nutrition of their children. Participants identified the availability of milk as a key factor. They noted that the health and nutrition of livestock, as well as the seasonal migration of livestock, which took them away from young children, were major factors affecting this availability.

The project therefore aimed to improve the food security and nutritional status of children by addressing these factors and improving the milk production system. It maintained the health of livestock by providing supplementary feed, vaccinations and de-worming as well as ensuring the availability of a sufficient water supply.

Results from the Milk Matters evaluation (Sadler *et al*., 2012), carried out by Save the Children in collaboration with Tufts University, found that milk availability and consumption by young children improved in the intervention sites relative to the control sites. By the end of the intervention, 90 percent of the children in Waruf were given milk, compared with only 31 percent in the control region, Fadhato.

Where the intervention worked well and intervention coverage of households was high, the increase in milk consumption seen (1 050 ml/day compared with 650 ml/day in the control site) translated into an additional 264 kcal of energy, 12.8 g of protein and considerably higher intakes of essential fatty acids, vitamins and minerals per child each day. For a two-year-old child this increase in nutrient intake would meet around 26 percent of energy and 98 percent of protein requirements.

Nutritional impacts were seen in the intervention sites. During a severe drought, the nutritional status of children in the intervention sites remained stable while it deteriorated significantly in non-intervention sites during the period of the programme.

This intervention improved nutritional outcomes for children, while at the same time enabling families to retain key assets (in the form of livestock) during a period in which significant risks to food and nutrition security unfolded. The project shows that food production systems, including pastoralist husbandry, can be shaped so that they enhance household livelihoods and simultaneously lead to improvements in child nutrition.

Source: Contributed by Save the Children (UK).

Evidence shows that HFP programmes in Bangladesh have improved food security for almost 5 million vulnerable people in diverse agro-ecological zones. There is convincing evidence of HFP's impact on household production, improved dietary quality and intake of micronutrient-rich foods, but neither improvements in actual micronutrient status nor the cost-effectiveness of the approach have been fully demonstrated (Iannotti, Cunningham and Ruel, 2009).

A recent review of household food production strategies and their effect on nutrition by Girard *et al.* (2012) notes that many factors determine the effectiveness of such strategies in influencing nutritional outcomes. For one, when infectious disease is common, additional interventions are needed as the impacts of production strategies will be limited. The review also found that the impacts of production strategies are difficult to discern because it is hard to establish how much of the additional output is sold and how much of the food consumed at home is consumed by women and children. The authors concluded that the existing evidence, although scarce, indicates that production strategies can improve intakes of micronutrient-rich foods by women and young children when they have clear nutrition objectives and integrate nutrition education and gender considerations.

In Viet Nam, the VAC (Vuon, Ao, Chuong – Crop farming, Aquaculture, Animal husbandry) system is one such integrated approach that seems to have produced positive effects on nutrition. The VAC system typically includes: a pond stocked with fish placed close to the home; livestock or poultry pens situated near or over the pond to provide an immediate source of organic fertilization; and gardens that include both annual and perennial crops for year-round food provision and products for market. Viet Nam's National Nutrition Survey 2000 showed marked improvements from 1987 in terms of animal-source foods and fruit and vegetable consumption. Although this progress is due to multiple factors, VAC is considered to have played an important role (Hop, 2003). As a result, the prevalence of child malnutrition and chronic energy deficiency in women of reproductive age decreased and there was a substantial increase in the incomes and the health and nutrition of Vietnamese rural populations (Hop, 2003).

As suggested above, production projects are more likely to succeed when gender roles are taken into account in project design and implementation (Berti, Krasevec and Fitzgerald, 2004; Quisumbing and Pandolfelli, 2010). Implementation modalities are important (Kumar and Quisumbing, 2011). Gender-specific time constraints are particularly important. Strategies that place new time demands on women can reduce the time available for breastfeeding, child care, food preparation and fetching water – all of which are related to nutrition. New time demands can also reduce the time available to cultivate nutrient-dense foods in kitchen gardens or acquire such food from the market. Policies and projects that make productivity-enhancing, time-saving technologies and approaches for activities traditionally undertaken by women, such as fetching water and firewood, weeding, hoeing, food processing and local marketing of produce, can significantly enhance the nutrition of women and children (Herforth, Jones and Pinstrup-Andersen, 2012; Kes and Swaminathan, 2006; Gill *et al.*, 2010).

Making food more nutritious

Poor households' diets typically rely on a single starchy staple to provide the bulk of energy consumed. Non-staple foods that are high in micronutrients – such as milk, eggs, fish, meat, fruits and vegetables – are often too expensive for the poor to purchase in adequate quantities. Dietary diversity is often a luxury that the poor cannot afford. Several approaches seek to enhance the diversity of the foods that the poor themselves produce.

Agronomic practices to improve nutrition

Improving the fertility of soils through the use of organic or inorganic fertilizers containing balanced concentrations of nitrogen, potassium and phosphorous can enhance crop yields and improve the micronutrient concentrations in crops. Adding specific micronutrients to fertilizers or irrigation water can further enhance yields and micronutrient concentrations.

Adding micronutrients to soils in the Indian states of Andhra Pradesh, Madhya Pradesh and Rajasthan enhanced yields by 20–80 percent and a further 70–120 percent when micronutrients were added in conjunction with nitrogen and phosphorous (Dar, 2004). These results were found for a number of crops, including maize, sorghum, greengram, pigeonpea, castor, chickpea, soybean and wheat. Yield increases achieved through balanced crop fertilization can reduce the land area needed to grow staple crops and thus add to the sustainability of the farming system.

Additions of iodine, in the form of potassium iodate, to irrigation water have been used to eliminate iodine deficiency in villages in northwestern China (Cao *et al.*, 1994; Ren *et al.*, 2008). A single application of iodine to the farmers' fields corrected iodine deficiencies in villagers consuming the crops grown on these fields for at least four years at a low cost of around US$0.05 per person per year. Livestock productivity also improved by around 30 percent because livestock in the region had previously been iodine-deficient.

Dietary zinc deficiencies can also be addressed through the use of micronutrient fertilizers in rice production, although complementary interventions such as plant selection, breeding local varieties for zinc content and changing cooking methods are also beneficial (Mayer *et al.*, 2011). The authors conclude that these changes, taken together, could potentially double the zinc content of rice and increase children's total dietary zinc intake by more 50 percent.

While micronutrient-enriched fertilizer is a promising technology, both in terms of nutritional efficacy and economic efficiency, several challenges have so far limited its adoption by farmers. Assessing micronutrient availability in soils is complex, and there is a lack of quantitative data on the micronutrient density of food crops grown on different types of soil (Nubé and Voortman, 2011).

Farmers must perceive an incentive to use micronutrient fertilizers either in the form of nutritional benefits or economic benefits such as higher yields or a market premium for the product. Because most micronutrients are not readily visible to consumers, farmers would be unlikely to receive a premium in the absence of effective education, marketing and labelling campaigns. Governments that already provide incentives for fertilizer use might consider including micronutrient fertilizers as their nutritional effects offer clear public good benefits that represent an investment in human capital.

Biofortification through plant breeding

Biofortification is a nutrition-specific intervention designed to enhance the micronutrient content of foods through the use of agronomic practices and plant breeding. Unlike food fortification, which occurs during food processing (discussed in Chapter 4), biofortification involves enriching the micronutrient content of plants. Biofortification can benefit farm households that produce primarily for their own consumption, as well as urban and rural households that purchase biofortified foods (Bouis *et al.*, 2011).

Plant breeders typically consider a range of objectives in developing a new crop variety, such as yield, disease resistance, processing characteristics and cooking qualities. In the process of biofortification, breeders give relatively higher priority to nutritional content among these objectives.

Biofortification through plant breeding can involve conventional varietal selection and breeding or more advanced molecular biology techniques such as marker-assisted selection or genetic engineering. Breeders can use the existing genetic diversity in a crop species and its wild relatives to identify, select and breed varieties that have higher nutritional content. Where a nutritional trait does not exist within the genome of the target crop, genetic engineering can be used to introduce the trait from another species. Biofortification programmes typically focus on staple grains or tubers and are aimed at smallholder farmers, although biofortified crops can also be cultivated by large-scale commercial farmers.

Biofortified crops can entail high start-up costs in the form of research, development and dissemination, but once biofortified staples are integrated into the food chain, they continue to provide micronutrient intervention with little additional input (Qaim, Stein and Meenakshi, 2007). In 2008, biofortification interventions were ranked the fifth most cost-effective development intervention by the Copenhagen Consensus (2008).

The Consultative Group on International Agricultural Research (CGIAR) programme HarvestPlus carries out extensive R&D on biofortification, relying on conventional plant breeding.[16] Starting in 2003, HarvestPlus has been developing and delivering biofortified staples in countries with populations most at risk of micronutrient deficiencies. Table 2 lists the expected release years for various biofortified crops being developed by the HarvestPlus programme. Widespread adoption is expected to take another decade.

The most promising results so far have been achieved with orange-fleshed sweet potato (OFSP). Unlike the typical white and yellow sweet potato varieties produced in Southern Africa, orange varieties are rich in vitamin A. HarvestPlus selected and adapted

[16] See HarvestPlus (2011) for more details.

TABLE 2
Biofortified staple food crops implemented by the HarvestPlus programme and actual or expected release year

BIOFORTIFIED CROP	MICRONUTRIENT	COUNTRY OF FIRST RELEASE	AGRONOMIC TRAIT	YEAR
Sweet potato	Provitamin A	Mozambique, Uganda	Disease resistance, drought tolerance, acid soil tolerance	2007
Cassava	Provitamin A	Democratic Republic of the Congo, Nigeria	Disease resistance	2011
Bean	Iron, zinc	Democratic Republic of the Congo, Rwanda	Virus resistance, heat and drought tolerance	2012
Maize	Provitamin A	Zambia	Disease resistance, drought tolerance	2012
Pearl millet	Iron, zinc	India	Mildew resistance, drought tolerance, disease resistance	2012
Rice	Iron, zinc	Bangladesh, India	Disease and pest resistance, cold and submergence tolerance	2013
Wheat	Iron, zinc	India, Pakistan	Disease and lodging resistance	2013

Note: HarvestPlus also supports biofortification of banana/plantain (vitamin A), lentil (iron, zinc), potato (iron, zinc) and sorghum (iron, zinc).
Source: Modified from Bouis *et al.*, 2011.

orange-fleshed varieties grown in Northern America to suit the agronomic conditions found in Southern Africa and introduced them to more than 24 000 households in Mozambique and Uganda. Beyond plant breeding, the programme worked closely with farmers and consumers to ensure compatibility with consumer preferences and to promote behaviour change and dissemination. Many existing sweet potato farmers switched to the orange variety from yellow or white varieties, and many others were new to cultivating sweet potatoes.

The OFSP intervention in both countries significantly increased vitamin A intake among children and women in the relevant households (Hotz, *et al.*, 2012). In Uganda, this was associated with a lower likelihood of vitamin A deficiency among children and women. At follow-up, the OFSP was found to be the dominant source of vitamin A in the diet, providing 80 percent of total vitamin A intake among reference children (Hotz *et al.*, 2011).

Questions remain about the readiness of consumers to purchase biofortified foods, especially when they look or taste different from traditional varieties. Receptivity is likely to vary depending on the crop and trait, local tastes and preferences, and the breeding technique. Early evidence regarding OFSP suggests that consumers are willing to buy them and may even pay a premium. In Uganda, consumers are willing to pay as much for the orange-fleshed varieties of sweet potato as for the white varieties even in the absence of a promotional campaign, and they are willing to pay a significant premium when provided with information about their nutritional benefits (Chowdury *et al.*, 2011). Similar results were found for nutritionally enhanced orange maize in Zambia, where consumers did not confuse it with ordinary yellow or white maize and were willing to pay a premium when its introduction was accompanied by nutrition information (Meenakshi *et al.*, 2012).

Success in introducing and establishing biofortified crops will be helped by understanding gender roles in production, consumption and marketing of these foods (Bouis and Islam, 2012a). Women's role as caregivers and in food preparation may make them particularly receptive to foods that have specific health attributes. In Uganda, OFSP uptake has been encouraged for health and nutrition reasons, which may have contributed to making women more likely to grow these varieties on the parcels they control (Gilligan *et al.*, 2012). Bouis and Islam (2012a, p. 2) report that "a key factor in the success of OFSP was the critical role played by women, both as caregivers of young children and as producers and retailers of OFSP".

Genetic engineering is being used to enhance the vitamin and mineral content and bioavailability of some staple crops where these traits are not available within the target crop genome (Waters and Sankaran, 2011; White and Broadley, 2009). Research is under way on nutrients such as vitamins A and E, riboflavin, folic acid, iron and zinc. The best-known example is "Golden Rice", which was developed by the Golden Rice Network, an international consortium of public research institutions, and is currently undergoing pre-market testing.

The potential of biofortified crops is high but, with the exception of OFSP, their nutritional efficacy and sustainability have not yet been well established. In response to this, HarvestPlus partners are studying these issues with regard to biofortified beans, pearl millet, wheat, rice, cassava and maize. The first round of findings should be available in 2013 (Bouis and Islam, 2012b).

Conclusions and key messages

Agricultural production and productivity growth support nutritional outcomes through their traditional roles of generating incomes for populations that depend on the sector for their livelihoods and by making food more available and accessible for all consumers. Agricultural productivity growth makes food more sustainable by reducing the resources required for production. If research priorities focus more closely on integrated production systems and nutrient-dense fruits, vegetables, legumes and livestock products, then agricultural production can contribute more to making food more diverse and nutritious.

Agricultural productivity growth depends on the existence of an enabling policy and institutional environment – good governance, macroeconomic stability, rural infrastructure, secure property rights (especially for women) and effective market institutions (FAO, 2012b). Agricultural R&D is necessary to maintain productivity growth but also to improve the diversity, sustainability and nutritional quality of the food supply.

Agricultural support policies could be more conducive to better nutrition by rebalancing support to favour healthier, more sustainable diets. Current policies have fewer nutritional impacts than they could if they included nutrition among their primary objectives.

Key messages

- Agricultural production contributes to better nutrition by making food more available and accessible. The traditional roles of agricultural production and productivity growth in generating incomes and reducing food prices will continue to be of crucial importance in the coming decades. At the same time, the sector can and must do more to improve the sustainability, diversity and nutritional quality of food.
- Agricultural production policies should focus on creating an enabling environment and allowing market signals to encourage production. Agricultural R&D priorities must continue to include the sustainable intensification of staple food production, but must also be made more nutrition-sensitive, with a stronger focus on nutrient-dense foods such as legumes, fruits, vegetables and animal-source foods. Greater efforts must be directed towards interventions that diversify smallholder production, such as integrated farming systems. Efforts to raise the micronutrient content of staples directly through biofortification are particularly promising. Agricultural interventions are more likely to be successful in improving nutrition when they are combined with nutrition education and implemented with sensitivity to gender roles.
- A substantial body of evidence supports the crucial role of agriculture in improving nutrition, but the causal relationships are complex. Agricultural interventions generally have multiple objectives such as productivity growth, cropping diversity or income generation, and their impacts on nutrition are often indirect and dynamic. As a result, their impacts are more difficult to evaluate accurately than simple medical interventions. Ultimately, however, agricultural interventions will be much more effective as they lead to a virtuous cycle of growth, poverty reduction, improved nutrition and better health.

4. Food supply chains for better nutrition[17]

Agricultural products reach consumers through food supply chains. Each link in a food supply chain affects the availability, affordability, diversity and nutritional quality of foods. How foods are handled throughout a chain influences their nutritional content and prices as well as the ease with which consumers can access them. This, in turn, shapes consumer choices, dietary patterns and nutritional outcomes.

Opportunities exist at each link in the chain to deliver more diverse and nutritious foods. For example, proper household storage can preserve nutrients; food processors can use more nutritious inputs or can fortify foods during processing; logistics firms can employ nutrient-preserving techniques for storage and transport; and retailers can provide a more diverse range of foods consistently throughout the year. At every link in the chain, better technologies and management practices can preserve nutrients, reduce food losses and waste, and enhance efficiency and lower prices for nutritious foods.

This chapter reviews (i) transformations in traditional and modern food supply chains and the general impact pathways through which supply chains influence nutritional outcomes and (ii) specific opportunities to improve nutritional performance throughout the supply chain, including improving efficiency, reducing nutrient waste and losses and enhancing the nutritional quality of foods.

Transformation of food supply chains

Food supply chains are changing in complex ways, driven by economic development, urbanization and social change and facilitated in many cases by policy reforms. Modern supply chains led by large food processors, distributors and retailers are expanding rapidly in many developing countries, where they may complement rather than replace traditional supply chains. Modern supply chains exist alongside and integrate to varying degrees with traditional supply chains such as farmer/traders, wet markets, small independent stores and street vendors (Gómez and Ricketts, 2012). At the same time, traditional farmers' markets are re-emerging in many developed countries to satisfy consumer preferences for local, seasonal and artisanal products. The result is great diversity in the way food is supplied to consumers.

Supply chains differ according to the country context, the location and characteristics of producers and consumers, and the goods themselves (e.g. fresh produce, dairy products or processed goods). Some of the modern food companies are international in scope and operate global procurement and distribution activities, although many are national or regional food companies that have emerged in Africa, Asia and Latin America and the Caribbean.

The increased industrialization of the food system has been accompanied by rapid consolidation and increasing integration of the different segments of the food industry (Reardon and Timmer, 2012). This consolidation is also cross-boundary, with multinational food companies investing heavily in developing countries over the last few decades. International food companies are major investors, producers and retailers in developing countries, but international trade comprises only 10 percent of total processed food sales, meaning that 90 percent of processed foods are produced domestically (Regmi and Gehlhar, 2005).

There is a high degree of market concentration in the food manufacturing and food retail sectors globally and in many countries (Stuckler and Nestle, 2012). This has raised concerns about the power of food companies over prices and also, increasingly,

[17] This chapter is based in part on Gómez and Ricketts (2012).

over the types of product marketed, the intensity of marketing and changes in local food cultures (Monteiro and Cannon, 2012).

Traditional and modern supply chains for different foods

In the traditional food systems of most developing countries, consumers in rural and urban areas typically buy most of their food from small independent retailers. Meat, fish, fruits, vegetables and bulk grains are typically sold in "wet markets" at roadside stands and open markets, while processed goods such as pasta, rice, packaged and canned items and some meat and dairy products are sold in small shops or kiosks. Fresh produce usually comes from farms in relatively close proximity to these markets and generally reflects local and seasonal production. Packaged and processed goods may be produced nationally or imported.

Multiple links connect producers to consumers through intricate networks. Numerous traders, wholesalers, retailers and other intermediaries procure products from local markets or directly from farmers and then channel them to the next link in the chain. Traditional market systems can include large regional markets that function like distribution hubs as well as smaller, local, weekly markets with a more limited range of products. Goods ripple out from these markets to smaller retailers in both urban and rural areas (Reardon, Henson and Gulati, 2010; Reddy, Murthy and Meena, 2010; Gorton, Sauer and Supatpongkul, 2011; Ruben *et al.*, 2007).

As the food system transforms, wet markets (including those for fish and meat as well as other fresh produce) may continue to be prevalent, but larger stores with a wider range of goods may replace the smaller kiosks. Production, purchasing and processing units all tend to increase in scale. Agribusiness input suppliers, food processors and retailers drive the integration of these activities, each of which may manage its own procurement and distribution activities. Supermarket chains begin to appear, often linked to foreign investors. They bring with them new technologies, more integrated supply chains and often greater links to their own suppliers outside the country. Although supermarkets establish themselves first in the largest cities, they subsequently spread to secondary cities (Reardon and Timmer, 2012).

Diverse supply chains for diverse diets

Despite the growth of supermarkets, traditional food systems are still the main avenue through which people in developing countries purchase most of their food. Even in those developing countries where supermarkets emerged earliest and have penetrated most, they control only about 50–60 percent of food retail. In most developing countries, including China and India, the spread of supermarkets started later and the corresponding food retail share is below 50 percent (Reardon and Gulati, 2008). Traditional retail outlets continue to be the preferred avenue for most consumers to access fresh, unprocessed products, such as fruits and vegetables (Figure 8). In Kenya, Nicaragua and Zambia, over 90 percent of all fruits and vegetables are purchased through traditional outlets.

At the same time, sales of processed and packaged foods are growing quickly in developing countries (Figure 9), and this growth is likely to continue. Evidence indicates that even low-income consumers buy processed and packaged foods in supermarkets (Cadilhon, Moustier and Poole, 2006; Goldman, Ramaswami and Krider, 2002), but, more interestingly, much of this growth is being fuelled by modern global food manufacturers selling products through traditional outlets in both urban and rural areas (Euromonitor, 2011a). In India, for example, small independent grocers called *kirana* stores, ubiquitous in urban and rural areas, sold over 53 percent of packaged foods at the retail level in 2010. The figure for similar outlets in Brazil, called *mercadinhos*, was over 21 percent (Euromonitor, 2011a). Between 1996 and 2002, while retailing of packaged foods in high-income countries grew by only 2.5 percent in per capita terms, it grew by 28 percent in lower-middle income countries and 12 percent in low-income countries (Hawkes *et al.*, 2010).

These examples show that aspects of traditional and modern systems exist in parallel and that the transformation of food systems is not a simple linear transformation from one to the other. In fact, integration between modern and traditional channels is often a key part of a corporate strategy. Following a successful business model used in Eastern Europe and in Latin America

FIGURE 8
Modern and traditional retail outlet shares of fresh fruit and vegetable market in selected countries

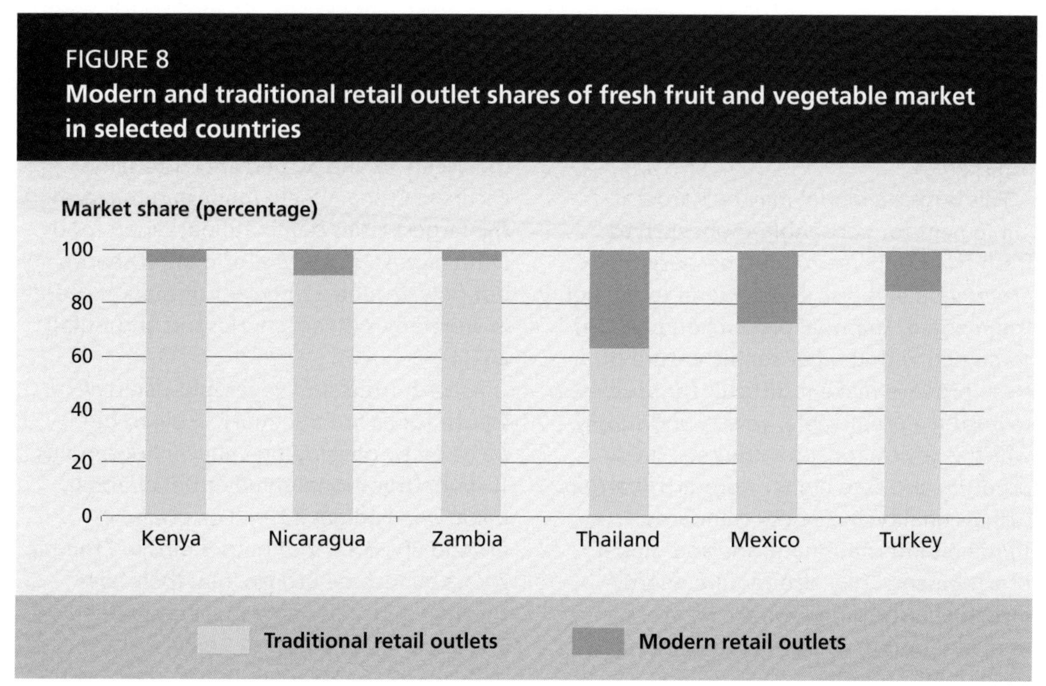

Notes: Countries are presented in ascending order of GDP per capita according to World Bank (2008) figures.
Sources: Kenya and Zambia: Tschirley *et al.*, 2010; Nicaragua and Mexico: Reardon, Henson and Gulati, 2010; Thailand: Gorton, Sauer and Supatpongkul, 2011; Turkey: Bignebat, Koc and Lemelilleur, 2009.

FIGURE 9
Retail sales of packaged food, by region

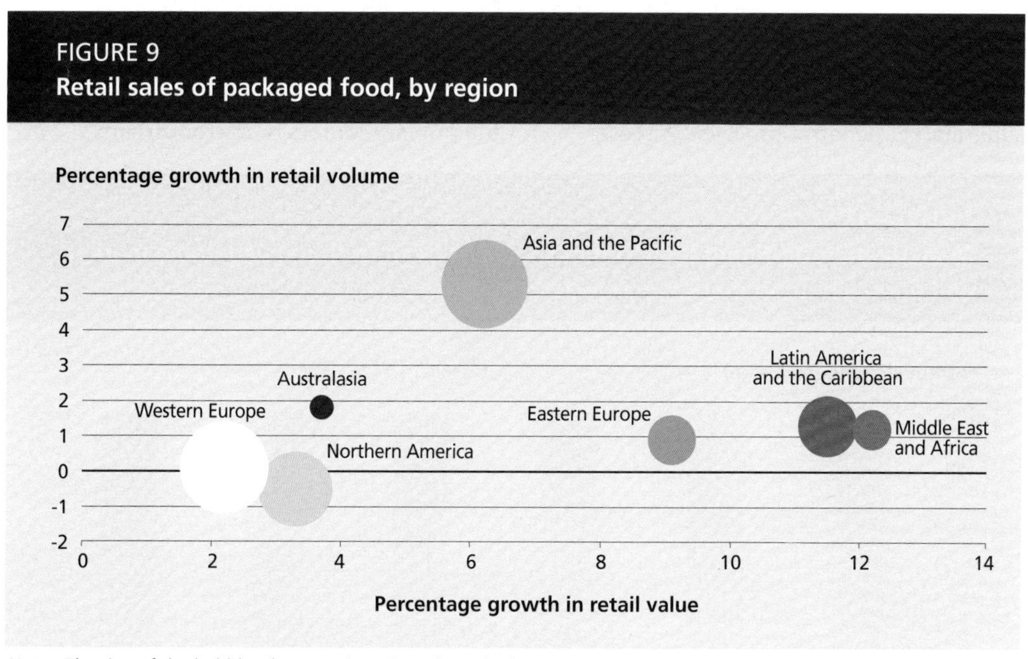

Notes: The size of the bubbles denotes the value of retail sales in US dollars for 2011 at fixed 2011 exchange rates and prices. The market values range from US$40.7 million in Australasia to US$581.6 million in Western Europe. Percentage growth refers to the period 2010–11.
Source: Authors' compilation using data supplied by Euromonitor.

and the Caribbean, major importers and supermarkets use packaged goods to link to traditional retailers and form mini-hubs for their products across the country. Over time, they increase their knowledge of local markets and leverage their brands to increase market share. Later, they expand into high-value fruit, vegetable, dairy and meat product categories (Hawkes *et al.*, 2010; Gorton, Sauer and Supatpongkul, 2011; Tschirley *et al.*, 2010; McKinsey, 2007; Minten and Reardon, 2008). Reardon and Timmer (2007) describe this business model in terms of waves, whereby supermarkets first enter certain product categories (processed and packaged goods), geographies (urban areas first) and socio-economic segments (high-income consumers) before expanding in other areas.

This business model may be harder to implement for perishable foods such as fresh fruits and vegetables, because their production and distribution tend to be highly fragmented. Seasonal production patterns combined with the perishable nature of fresh produce make it difficult for businesses to ensure a predictable, year-round supply, which is critical for supermarkets. These products also face higher non-tariff barriers, such as quality and safety standards, that limit international trade and global procurement. They also require energy-intensive distribution infrastructure, such as refrigeration, which is often lacking in developing countries.

The market shares accruing to modern and traditional vendors in the fresh fruit and vegetable and packaged foods markets appear to support this analysis. Figure 10 shows statistics from Mexico, Thailand and Turkey, all countries with high modern supermarket penetration. Even in these countries, traditional vendors have a larger share than modern ones in sales of fresh fruits and vegetables (around 60–85 percent), while the reverse is true for packaged foods (between 40 and 50 percent). The same occurs in China, where modern retailers in the largest cities dominate packaged foods (with almost 80 percent of market share), but only around 22 percent of market share in vegetables (Reardon, Henson and Gulati, 2010).

As with fruits and vegetables, animal-source foods are also more likely to be accessed by developing-country households through traditional retail outlets (Jabbar, Baker and Fadiga, 2010). For example, around 90 percent of households in Ethiopia, across all income groups, buy their beef through a local butcher in a wet market. The situation is similar in Kenya (camel milk, meat), Bangladesh (meat, dairy) and Viet Nam (pork), with traditional shops still the predominant location for purchase, especially for low-income households (Jabbar, Baker and Fadiga, 2010). These traditional outlets, therefore, seem to be the primary point of purchase for foods that are the primary sources of micronutrients.

FIGURE 10
Modern and traditional retail outlet shares of fresh fruit and vegetable market and packaged food market in selected countries

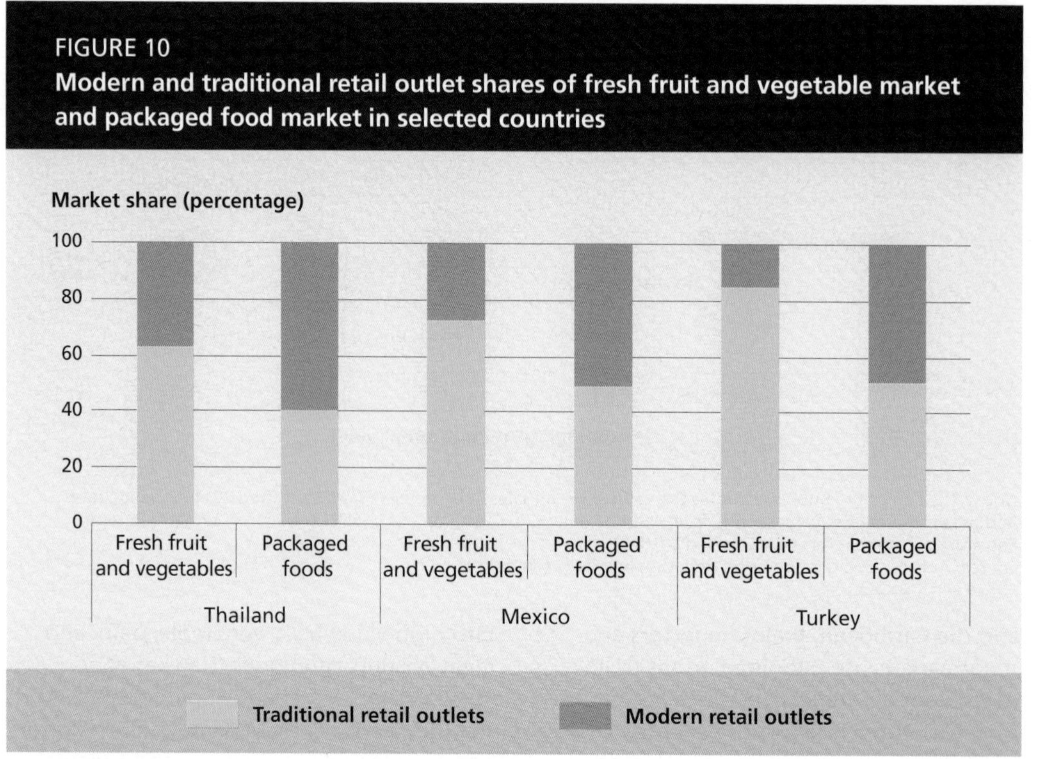

Note: Packaged foods include breakfast foods as well as preserved, canned, frozen and other ready-to-consume items. Countries are presented in ascending order of GDP per capita according to World Bank (2008) figures.
Sources: Euromonitor, 2012 and 2011b; and Gorton, Sauer and Supatpongkul, 2011.

Traditional outlets also continue to be important for sales of staples, which contribute a large part of energy requirements. In Kenya and Zambia, traditional retail outlets account for 60 percent or more of staple sales, even in urban areas (Jayne *et al.*, 2010).

Despite the rise of modern supply chains, traditional supply chains are still important for certain products and to certain types of consumer. The advantages of traditional outlets, particularly with respect to perishable products, appear to arise from three main interconnecting factors: ability to offer products at low prices, considerable flexibility in product standards, and convenience for consumers due to flexible retail market locations (Schipmann and Qaim, 2010; Wanyoike *et al.*, 2010; Jabbar and Admassu, 2010; Minten, 2008).

Traditional retailers typically operate under structures that give them pricing advantages relative to modern supermarkets. Lower labour and overhead costs, as well as higher product turnover rates, result in lower per-unit costs. Modern supermarkets need to provide additional services (e.g. processing, sorting, re-packing, refrigeration) and control significant physical assets (e.g. buildings and equipment), which add to their costs (Goldman, Ramaswami and Krider, 2002).

These differences in cost structure appear to allow traditional retailers to develop flexible pricing strategies for different locations and different socio-economic groups. Low-income consumers in Thailand and Viet Nam overwhelmingly purchase fruits and vegetables in traditional retail outlets because of lower prices (Mergenthaler, Weinberger and Qaim, 2009; Lippe, Seens and Isvilanonda, 2010). Modern supermarkets in Thailand charge significantly higher prices than traditional outlets, even controlling for differences in product quality (Schipmann and Qaim, 2011). On the other hand, in Chile food prices in wet markets were found to be higher than those in supermarkets in higher-income neighbourhoods while the opposite was true in low-income neighbourhoods in the same city (Dirven and Faiguenbaum, 2008). Price differences between modern and traditional outlets cannot be explained simply by the relevant processing and distribution model, but can also be linked to the economic landscape surrounding the store.

Product standards and consumer expectations for traditional food value chains may also be different, permitting the marketing of foods that modern supermarkets would reject and allowing traditional outlets to lower their prices. Evidence shows that all consumers care about quality but that those who frequent traditional outlets may have different priorities than those shopping at modern retail outlets. In Madagascar, consumers purchasing from traditional retailers considered meat type and smell highly important rather than other characteristics typically valued by supermarket buyers, such as origin, date of slaughter, fat content and whether or not the product had been under constant refrigeration (Minten, 2008). Supermarket prices, especially for fresh produce and livestock, may be higher than those in traditional outlets, making micronutrient-rich foods available in supermarkets less affordable for the poor (Dolan and Humphrey, 2000; Schipmann and Qaim, 2011; Reddy, Murthy and Meena, 2010).

At the same time, proximity and convenience are major factors affecting decisions about where to shop, especially in urban areas where more choice exists (Zameer and Mukherjee, 2011; Tschirley *et al.*, 2010; Neven *et al.*, 2005; Jabbar and Admassu, 2010). Both of these factors are key advantages of traditional retailers. Small independent shops often proliferate in low-income areas, even if product selection is limited. Traditional retailers may also be more able to respond to the purchasing constraints of the poor and offer smaller, affordable quantities of goods and provide customers with shop credit if needed.

In any case, the location of traditional and modern outlets does seem to be associated with income levels. Traditional outlets are more likely to be located in low-income areas and so meet demand from low-income consumers. In contrast, modern value chains appear to be located where they can provide access to mostly urban, higher-income households. In Kenya and Zambia, for example, modern supermarkets mostly serve households in the top 20 percent of the income range (Tschirley *et al.*, 2010).

Traditional retailers also appear to be able to respond better to the demand for food from people living in more remote rural locations, regardless of their income level. This is likely to remain the case until improved roads make travel to urban areas, with their greater variety of products, easier and less time-consuming.

The coexistence of traditional and modern supply chains appears to support the availability of diverse, affordable diets for a variety of different consumers. By providing convenient access to micronutrient-rich foods at a range of price and quality combinations, traditional food outlets can support lower-income consumers in purchasing nutritious foods.

Supply chain transformation and nutrition

As the discussion above shows, a multiplicity of food options are available to today's consumers. Consumers in both urban and rural areas in developing countries still seem to favour traditional outlets (e.g. small shops, open markets) for perishable items such as fruits and vegetables, fish and meat. Supermarkets tend to be associated with urban, higher-income areas while low-income consumers, in both urban and rural areas, still do most of their shopping at traditional retailers. Consumers favour supermarkets for processed and packaged goods, although traditional outlets are also important retailers of packaged goods.

Nutritionally, the result is that traditional retail outlets are the primary place for poor consumers to access fresh foods rich in micronutrients as well as packaged goods. Interventions that can help shape nutritional outcomes through the traditional retail sector are those that can lower prices by making the supply chain more efficient and reducing waste. Better infrastructure and market access for smallholder fruit, vegetable and livestock producers can increase the diversity of foods available in rural and urban markets.

The increased availability of packaged and processed goods in traditional as well as modern retail outlets can increase the availability of energy for low-income consumers. However, such foods are often high in sugar, fats and salt and low in important micronutrients, and there is a risk that consumers could potentially replace other important elements of a diverse diet, such as fruits and vegetables, with these products. As a result, micronutrient deficiencies could potentially continue even as energy intake increases. Poorer diets could combine with other factors (such as changes in life style, reduced manual labour) and lead to increases in overweight and obesity (Harris and Graff, 2012; Garde, 2008; Caballero, 2007).

Some argue that modern value chain processors and retailers could develop products with improved nutritional characteristics, such as micronutrient fortification or reduced trans-fats. Public–private partnerships can play an important role when they facilitate the development of more nutritious foods by food manufacturers and their subsequent distribution through traditional retailers (World Economic Forum, 2009; Wojcicki and Heyman, 2010).

This analysis underscores the complexity of the transformation that supply chains are currently undergoing. Optimal diets are not a guaranteed outcome. But supply chains can be shaped to improve nutrition. In tandem with economic development and the nutrition transition, policies, programmes and investments should seek to take advantage of the transformation process to encourage provision of adequate, but not excessive, amounts of energy and of a high-quality, varied diet with sufficient micronutrients.

Enhancing nutrition through food supply chains

The discussion so far provides an insight into the types of supply chain that exist and how they channel different foods from producer to consumer. This is helpful for understanding the entry points where interventions could be used to improve nutrition. This section presents some examples and evidence of measures that can improve the nutritional performance of supply chains, including through improving their overall efficiency in enhancing the availability and accessibility of a wide diversity of foods, reducing post-harvest nutrient losses and improving the nutritional quality of foods through fortification and reformulation.

Improving supply chain efficiency

Raising the efficiency of supply chains can help meet the simultaneous challenge of lowering the costs of food to consumers and increasing the revenue of supply chain participants. Both lower prices (for consumers) and higher incomes (for smallholders and other producers) support the possibility of improving nutrition through a more adequate and varied diet.

Companies driving the transformation of modern food systems seek greater integration through vertical coordination of primary producers, input suppliers and processors. Such integration seems to hold the greatest potential for livestock and other capital-intensive food products (Swinnen and Maertens, 2006; Kaplinsky and Morris, 2001; Gulati *et al.*, 2007; Burch and Lawrence, 2007; IFAD, 2003).

In an integrated system, consumer demand and product information flow upstream from retailers to suppliers, who make contractual arrangements with producers (Reardon and Barrett, 2000). These contracts may include provision of inputs, credit and technical and marketing assistance. This can enable farmers to increase their productivity and profits through better access to inputs and timely receipt of payments (Swinnen and Maertens, 2006). To ensure that farmers do benefit and that lower costs translate into lower prices, appropriate regulatory policies that ensure a competitive manufacturing and retail sector will also be required.

At the same time, integrated actions throughout a supply chain can improve the nutrient content of foods and nutritional outcomes for consumers (Box 8). Nutrition-enhancing actions within the food supply

BOX 8

Improving livelihoods and nutrition throughout the bean value chain

Women and men in East Africa typically cultivate small farms with variable soil fertility and erratic rainfall. They have limited access to high-quality seeds, advanced production and post-harvest technologies, credit, extension or training, all of which could help to improve yields and production and reduce post-harvest losses. Typically, even if these farmers could increase production, they are not well-linked to domestic and regional markets.

In Rwanda and Uganda, a partnership involving universities, research institutions and NGOs is addressing key points in the value chain for common beans. The goal is to improve food and nutrition security by improving production, linking producers to the market and increasing consumption of more nutritious foods. To improve bean yields and bean quality, the project focuses on improving management practices and technologies. In addition to improved production practices, this includes better techniques for harvesting, drying and storing beans.

To increase the nutritional value and appeal of the beans, researchers developed improved processing procedures (de-hulling, soaking, milling, fermentation, germination and extrusion). The digestibility and nutritional value of the beans was enhanced by reducing phytates and polyphenols that limit iron uptake. To increase consumption, the project developed bean-based, protein-rich composite flours for use in cooking and baking as well as a special weaning porridge. Additional research aims to produce and market a variety of bean-flour-based snacks.

Extension materials were developed to increase knowledge about bean production and utilization. Materials cover the basics of feeding children aged 6–59 months, methods of preparing beans that reduce cooking time and enhance nutrient bio-availability, as well as how to prepare bean-based composite flour and use it in making porridges, cakes, biscuits and bread.

Source: Contributed by Robert Mazur, Professor of Sociology and Associate Director for Socioeconomic Development, Center for Sustainable Rural Livelihoods, Iowa State University, United States of America.

chain are relevant for all households, urban and rural alike, because even rural dwellers in developing countries as diverse as Malawi, Nepal and Peru buy a third or more of their food via markets (Garrett and Ersado, 2003).

Integrating smallholders into domestic food value chains continues to pose challenges. Poor performance of other aspects of the value chain, such as storage, transport and distribution, can impede smallholder market participation. Investments in public goods that support the development of transport, communication and service infrastructure can substantially reduce producer risk, improve value chain performance and so raise smallholder income.

A study in Kenya showed that investments in infrastructure can reduce the significant marketing costs smallholders incur in delivering crops to buyers. If these costs, estimated at 15 percent of retail value, could be reduced, farmer earnings could be increased without driving up food prices (Renkow, Hallstrom and Karanja, 2004). Other programmes, such as a number of public–private partnerships, have improved overall market efficiency and smallholders' ability to engage with the market by using modern communication technologies to facilitate the flow of information (Aker, 2008; de Silva and Ratnadiwakara, 2005). Policies that support the development of financial markets in rural areas can also improve the ability of small- and medium-sized traders to purchase surplus production from smallholders (Coulter and Shepherd, 1995).

Reducing nutrient waste and losses

A recent FAO report estimates that roughly one-third of food produced globally for human consumption is lost or wasted (Gustavsson *et al.*, 2011). In addition to the quantitative food losses, qualitative losses also occur as nutrients deteriorate during storage, processing and distribution. Nutrient losses occur both during on-farm storage, preservation and preparation, and during later storage, processing and transport from farms to points of sale. Rodents, insects and microbial spoilage are the main reasons for loss and the underlying causes are limitations in techniques for harvesting, processing, preservation and storage; in methods of packaging and transportation; and in infrastructure, such as storage and cooling facilities. Food waste reduces the sustainability of food systems, as more production is required to feed the same number of people, which wastes seeds, fertilizer, irrigation water, labour, fossil fuels and other agricultural inputs (Floros *et al.*, 2010).

In developing countries, most losses occur at the farm level and along the supply chain, before arriving at the consumer. Gustavsson *et al.* (2011) found that only 5–15 percent of food losses occur at the consumer level in the developing regions considered, compared with 30–40 percent in the developed regions. The consumer share of food losses and waste can be very high in specific locations; for example, the amount of food wasted in one community in New York State in the United States of America in one year was sufficient to feed everyone in the community for 1.5 months and 60 percent of the losses occurred after the food was purchased by the consumer (Griffin, Sobal and Lyson, 2009).

With such large losses, reducing post-harvest losses could increase food supplies and reduce food prices significantly (assuming efforts to reduce waste generate greater benefits than their costs). This could potentially improve affordability and diversity. The losses of some micronutrient-rich foods such as fruits and vegetables and fish are typically greater than losses of cereals. Chadha *et al.* (2011) note that in Cambodia, Lao People's Democratic Republic and Viet Nam, about 17 percent of the vegetable crop is lost due to post-harvest problems. A study covering several sub-Saharan African countries concluded that losses in small-scale fisheries reached 30 percent or more. Losses were particularly high at the drying, packaging, storage and transportation stages, with key constraints related to poor fish-handling practices and outdated techniques and facilities (Akande and Diei-Quadi, 2010).

Post-harvest food losses disproportionately affect the poor, who have less capacity for food preservation and safe storage (Gómez *et al.*, 2011). At-home techniques for preservation, packaging, storage and preparation could be adapted to preserve nutrients (Box 9). Many effective

BOX 9
Food processing, preservation and preparation in the home and micronutrient intakes

The ways in which households process, preserve and cook food also contribute to micronutrient intakes as these activities affect the bioavailability of some key micronutrients. Traditional food-processing methods can enhance micronutrient availability (Gibson, Perlas and Hotz, 2006). Germination and malting can improve the bioavailability of iron by a factor of 8–12. Soaking grains and legumes, a fairly typical household practice, can remove anti-nutrients that inhibit iron absorption (Tontisirin, Nantel and Bhattacharjeef, 2002). Gibson and Hotz (2001) describe interventions that can enhance the content and bioavailability of micronutrients in a representative daily menu for rural Malawian preschoolers. For example, soaking maize flour used for maize porridges is one intervention that enhances the absorption of micronutrients.

Traditional food preservation techniques used in the home, such as sun-drying, canning and pickling of fruits and vegetables can enhance the bioavailability of micronutrients and preserve surplus micronutrient-rich foods for year-round use (Aworh, 2008; Hotz and Gibson, 2007). A long-term study in Malawi showed that a range of traditional strategies combined with promotion of micronutrient-rich foods resulted in improvements in both haemoglobin and lean body mass and a lower incidence of common infections (Hotz and Gibson, 2007). However, traditional processes can be time-consuming and labour-intensive and some such processes can result in *decreased* micronutrient availability (Lyimo *et al.*, 1991; Aworh, 2008).

Cooking using moderate heat and for short time periods as well as cooking closer to meal times, if possible, can help increase micronutrient bioavailability. For example, cooking green leafy vegetables with mild heat can increase the bioavailability of heat-sensitive nutrients such as vitamin C. Use of appropriate quantities of fat or oil in stir frying or similar methods can also increase micronutrient bioavailability, because oils facilitate absorption of certain nutrients (Tontisirin, Nantel and Bhattacharjeef, 2002).

interventions for reducing post-harvest losses are known (e.g. small-scale post-harvest storage facilities, improved pre-harvest management and/or increased food-processing opportunities); however, little is known about the impacts of such initiatives on nutrition (Silva-Barbeau *et al.*, 2005).

Enhancing the nutritional quality of foods

Fortification during processing is the most common means for improving the nutritional quality of foods.[18] Food companies can also reformulate processed foods to change the nutritional profile of the products offered. They frequently do so in response to consumer demand, for example, for foods with low-fat, low-carbohydrate, gluten-free or other nutritional attributes. Other than mandatory fortification, government policy has seldom directly influenced food reformulation for improved nutritional quality (such as reducing as trans-fats) beyond mandatory fortification.

Fortifying commonly consumed foods with specific key micronutrients can be an effective and economically efficient way to treat nutrition-related disorders. The Universal Salt Iodization initiative, which began in 1990, increased the proportion of the world's population with access to iodized salt from 20 percent to 70 percent by 2008, although iodine deficiency remains a public health problem in more than 40 countries (Horton, Mannar and Wesley, 2008). Most food fortification efforts

[18] Food fortification is "..the addition of one or more essential nutrients to a food whether or not it is normally contained in the food for the purpose of preventing or correcting a demonstrated deficiency of one or more nutrients in the population or specific population groups" (FAO and WHO, 1991).

BOX 10
The Grameen Danone Partnership

Groupe Danone, a multinational corporation, together with Grameen Bank, a Bangladeshi NGO known for expertise in micro-credit lending, founded Grameen Danone Foods (GDF) in 2006. Together with the Global Alliance for Improved Nutrition, GDF developed a yoghurt fortified with 30 percent of the recommended daily allowance (RDA) for zinc, iron, vitamin A and iodine and 12.5 percent of the RDA for calcium (Socialinnovator, 2012).

Beyond producing a fortified and nutritious yogurt targeted towards improving the nutritional needs of poor children in Bangladesh, the partnership also aimed to help the poor in the community by involving them in all stages of the value chain. The partnership set out to build up to 50 factories by 2020, with around 1 500 new jobs and 500 new milk producers associated with each factory. Although some of these goals have fallen short, there are currently up to 500 local women who sell yogurt throughout the Bogra district, making roughly US$30 per month. In addition, Rodrigues and Baker (2012) report that GDF has redesigned its plants to use milk supplied by nearby dairy farmers with five cows or fewer and who lack working refrigeration. This, in turn, is promoting local community growth in the small-scale dairy sector that once existed purely for subsistence.

GDF also now employs around 900 saleswomen, who account for about 20 percent of total sales, with the remainder generated by a network of small shops in provincial towns in the Rajshahi district and by supermarkets in Bangladesh's large cities, including Dhaka, Sylhet and Chittagong (Rodrigues and Baker, 2012).

involve key micronutrients such as vitamins A and D, iodine, iron[19] and zinc (Box 10). Condiments such as salt and soy sauce and staple foods like maize and wheat flours, as well as vegetable oils, are good candidates for fortification because they are widely consumed, and low-cost technologies can produce varieties that are acceptable to consumers (Darnton-Hill and Nalubola, 2002).

Fortified products need to reach micronutrient-deficient consumers through existing or newly established distribution channels. Based on the analysis above, traditional supply chains such as corner stores, wet markets and other small retail outlets are likely to be the most effective channels for reaching poor consumers. The companies typically involved in fortifying foods are often national and have well-established distribution and marketing networks that can effectively deliver products to urban and rural populations, although some fortification technologies are easily applied by small-scale processors who may be more effective in reaching remote populations (Horton, Mannar and Wesley, 2008).

Micronutrient fortification of staple foods and condiments is generally inexpensive and highly cost-effective. Salt iodization can reach 80–90 percent of a target population at an annual cost of approximately US$0.05 per person. Fortification of flour with iron can reach up to 70 percent of a target population for about US$0.12 per person. The costs of reaching the remaining population, often in remote areas, will be higher, but these hard-to-reach individuals may derive a proportionally higher benefit from fortification, as they are often poorer, with less-nutritious diets and less access to health care. Despite the low costs of fortification, consumer prices of fortified

[19] Some concerns have been expressed about the use of iron supplements, after some studies showed adverse effects when non-iron-deficient individuals received supplements in malarial areas. However, the doses of iron from the supplements were significantly higher than those delivered by fortification, even in populations with very high flour consumption. Expert reviews convened by WHO and UNICEF recommended iron fortification of staple foods, condiments and complementary foods even in areas affected by high malaria transmission rates because this avoids the need for preventive supplementation. Other reviews have found that fortification with appropriate levels of iron is also safe for the small proportion of people with clinical disorders relating to iron absorption and storage (Horton, Mannar and Wesley, 2008).

products such as iodized salt may be higher because such products are usually refined, packaged, branded and marketed in ways that add costs beyond those associated with fortification itself (Horton, Mannar and Wesley, 2008).

Fortification programmes entail a range of initial costs, including population-based needs assessments, trials to determine appropriate foods and micronutrient levels, industry start-up costs, development of appropriate communication and social marketing programmes, and capacity-building for public-sector regulation, enforcement, monitoring and evaluation. The incremental cost of flour fortification may be perceived by millers as significant if the market environment does not enable them to recover the cost because of factors such as low consumer demand for fortified products or government controls on the price of the product. When the incremental cost of fortification cannot be sustained by millers or passed directly to the consumer, governments may assist with subsidies or tax exemptions. In some cases, such costs have been partially subsidized by international support through organizations such as the Micronutrient Initiative and the Global Alliance for Improved Nutrition, as well as other donors (Horton, Mannar and Wesley, 2008).

At the same time, consumer demand for fortified foods can be strengthened through education and marketing campaigns. This may involve public–private partnerships that work through existing manufacturing and distribution associations and build on the existing marketing strategies of the member firms. In West Africa, for example, the NGO Helen Keller International is working with the Association of Edible Oil Producing Industries to educate consumers about the benefits of vitamin A and promote the use of fortified cooking oil (Helen Keller International, 2012). These promotional and education campaigns include strong in-store support for nutrition education.

Conclusions and key messages

Traditional and modern value chains play complementary roles in providing consumers in urban and rural areas with available, accessible, diverse and nutritious foods. Each offers distinct challenges and opportunities for improving the nutritional performance of food systems.

Traditional marketing channels deliver nutritional benefits to low-income residents in urban areas, where they enjoy cost and location advantages, and to rural residents who are largely missed by modern value chains. Traditional value chains are a good source of affordable, micronutrient-rich foods, but poor post-harvest storage and distribution infrastructure can lead to significant food losses and deterioration in nutritional quality. Traditional value chains suffer from seasonal shortages and high transaction costs that can offset their ability to offer low prices. Interventions to improve the efficiency of traditional food value chains can be effective in improving access to micronutrients, particularly among poor people.

In contrast, modern value chains tend to have more efficient distribution chains, with better year-round availability of a wide variety of foods. They increase the availability of highly processed packaged goods, which may contribute to problems of overweight and obesity. The ability of modern food manufacturers to distribute processed and packaged foods through traditional marketing channels allows them to reach remote rural areas and urban neighbourhoods where residents have little or no access to modern supermarkets. This may reduce undernutrition for poor rural and urban residents while increasing overnutrition for more affluent consumers. At the same time, the increased availability of processed and packaged goods offers opportunities for collaboration among food manufacturers, donors and governments to implement profitable and socially beneficial food fortification initiatives that target micronutrient deficiencies.

This analysis highlights the interactions between traditional and modern value chain participants and suggests the need for a more nuanced view of the links between food chains and nutrition. Two issues in particular warrant rigorous investigation. First, very little evidence exists regarding the contribution of different traditional and modern supply chains on micronutrient deficiencies. Second, very little is known about demand substitution effects among processed and packaged foods, staples, fruits, vegetables and livestock products, and about how consumers respond to changes in relative prices of these product categories.

Key messages

- Traditional and modern food supply chains are changing rapidly to provide consumers with a diverse range of foods. They tend to serve different population groups and specialize in different types of food, yet both offer challenges and opportunities for improving nutrition. Understanding how food supply chains are changing can help policy-makers target interventions more effectively.
- Traditional supply chains are the primary channel through which low-income consumers in urban and rural areas purchase food. Enhancing the efficiency of traditional value chains can promote better nutritional outcomes by improving access by low-income consumers to safe, nutrient-dense foods, such as fruits, vegetables and livestock products.
- Modern supply chains play an important role in preserving the nutritional content of food and increasing the year-round availability and affordability of a diverse range of foods. The growth of modern food processing and retailing facilitates the use of fortification to combat specific micronutrient deficiencies, but also increases the availability of highly processed, packaged goods that may contribute to overweight and obesity.
- Reducing food and nutrient losses and waste throughout the food system can make an important contribution to better nutrition and also relieve pressure on productive resources. In low-income countries, most food and nutrient losses occur before products reach the consumer, that is, at the farm level and during storage, processing and distribution. In high-income countries, most losses and waste occur at the consumer level.

5. Helping consumers achieve better nutrition

To improve nutritional outcomes, food systems need to provide consumers with abundant, affordable, diverse and nutritious foods, and consumers need to choose balanced diets that provide adequate but not excessive amounts of energy. Previous chapters have discussed ways to make food systems more supportive of food security and better nutrition. Nutrition-sensitive food systems can give consumers better options, but ultimately it is consumers who choose what they eat. What consumers choose to eat influences their own nutritional outcomes and sends signals back through the food system – to retailers, processors and producers – that shape both what is produced and how sustainably it is produced.

Consumers need adequate incomes and knowledge with which to make better nutritional choices. Even when adequate food is available, the poorest households or those hit by external shocks may need food-based assistance programmes to access the food they need. In households where income is not a significant constraint to good nutrition, poor food and lifestyle choices mean that malnutrition may persist in the form of micronutrient deficiencies, overweight and obesity. This suggests that additional measures – education and incentives – may be necessary to encourage households to choose more appropriate foods as part of a diverse, nutritious diet for all family members.

This chapter reviews (i) food-based assistance programmes, including general food subsidies; (ii) nutrition-specific incentives, such as targeted food subsidies and taxes aimed at influencing food choices; and (iii) nutrition education programmes, including formal training, public information campaigns, regulation of advertising and labelling and measures aimed at improving the local food environment. Evidence shows that many of these interventions can help people achieve better nutrition, but they are often more effective in combination than alone. Integrated programmes that improve the food environment, enhance consumer awareness and provide incentives for healthier eating can motivate the life-long behavioural changes necessary to ensure that everyone is well nourished.

Food assistance programmes for better nutrition[20]

Governments have long used food assistance programmes to guarantee access of vulnerable populations to adequate food.[21] Food assistance programmes may deliver food directly to recipients or improve their ability to access food through voucher programmes or cash transfers. They may be part of broader social protection policies or be aimed more narrowly at increasing food consumption. The programmes may be targeted at specific vulnerable populations or provide food access support to the general population. The traditional focus has been on the provision of a minimum ration of basic staple foods, but the overall nutritional impacts of food assistance programmes have not always been given adequate attention. This section focuses on ways in which such programmes can promote good nutritional outcomes.

General food assistance programmes

Many developing countries and international donors use general food assistance programmes to protect food-insecure

[20] This section is based on Lentz and Barrett (2012).

[21] Many different kinds of social protection programmes exist, with additional objectives beyond food assistance. For example, cash- or food-for-work schemes focus more on providing food as a means of alleviating poverty; conditional cash transfers seek mostly to build human capital; and emergency food assistance programmes focus more on halting hunger and deteriorations in nutritional status.

people. Food assistance transfers can be given in the form of food, vouchers or cash, or as subsidized prices for targeted groups or the general population. Food assistance programmes and general food subsidies often apply to starchy staples such as bread and rice and to energy-dense foods such as sugar and cooking oil. Thus, they can provide an essential safety net for food-insecure populations; at the same time, they can also lead to monotonous diets with excessive energy and inadequate micronutrient content.

The impact of food assistance programmes on food security and nutrition depends on a host of factors related to local context and programme design (Bryce *et al.*, 2008; Barrett and Lentz, 2010). No single programming approach can meet all objectives in all contexts, and trade-offs will be unavoidable. General food assistance programmes can be more supportive of good nutritional outcomes, but this means giving nutrition higher priority in programme design.

The form in which food assistance is provided has a direct impact on nutritional outcomes. The percentage of the transfer actually consumed by recipients as food varies according to its form: it is highest when the transfer is given in the form of food, lowest when given as cash and somewhere in between if vouchers are used (del Ninno and Dorosh, 2003; Ahmed *et al.*, 2010).

The form in which a food assistance transfer is given also influences the diversity of foods consumed. For example, providing staple foods may alleviate hunger and increase energy intake but may not address micronutrient deficiencies. Cash transfers tend to result in more diverse diets, as they give recipients more choice over the food basket. For similar reasons, vouchers have been linked to increased dietary diversity when compared with in-kind food distributions based on staples (Meyer, 2007). On the other hand, in-kind food and commodity-denominated vouchers can allow agencies to target specific food interventions, such as vitamin-fortified vegetable oil, biofortified beans or micronutrient powders (Ryckembusch *et al.*, 2013).

The nutritional quality of in-kind food assistance can be improved and could constitute a cost-effective means of improving nutritional outcomes for vulnerable populations. Improving the quality of food aid rations by, for example, substituting fortified milled grains for whole grains, improving the standard maize-soy and wheat-soy blends, and delivering the appropriate levels of vegetable oil could increase the costs of current emergency and development food aid projects by 6.6 percent, but the expected nutritional gains would outweigh these costs (Webb *et al.*, 2011).

Targeted food assistance programmes

Better targeting of vulnerable populations can improve the effectiveness and efficiency of transfers aimed at increasing food security and nutrition (Lentz and Barrett, 2007). Women tend to dedicate more of any social security transfer to food and child health care services than do men, making gender a good targeting criterion in many circumstances (Attanasio, Battistin and Mesnard, 2009; Barber and Gertler, 2010; Broussard, 2012). Food assistance programmes that have nutrition objectives frequently target vulnerable demographic groups.

Prenatal and early childhood

Prenatal and early childhood programmes are widely regarded as among the most effective food-based programmes. Such programmes can address the energy and micronutrient needs of children under 24 months and their mothers through the use of targeted vouchers, micronutrient supplements and improved complementary foods.[22] They are most effective when designed to meet local needs and local contexts.

One of the best-studied prenatal and early childhood food assistance interventions is the United States Supplemental Nutrition Program for Women, Infants, and Children (WIC), established in 1972 to improve the health status of women, infants and children. WIC seeks to affect the dietary quality and habits of participants by providing nutrition education and foods designed to meet the special nutritional needs of low-income pregnant women and mothers with children up to five years of age. Food vouchers

[22] "Complementary" feeding interventions are considered more suitable for treating and preventing moderate malnutrition, while "therapeutic" feeding interventions are suitable for treating severe malnutrition and are generally considered medical interventions (Horton *et al.*, 2010).

issued under the programme are limited to a list of foods with specific nutrients (protein, calcium, iron, vitamins A, B_6, C and D and folate). A summary of the vast literature evaluating WIC concludes that this combination of education plus vouchers "is associated with ... positive effects on child growth, improved dietary status, and greater access to and use of health care" (Devaney, 2007, p.16).

An increasingly common approach to addressing micronutrient deficiencies in early childhood is through distribution of multiple micronutrient powders. These powders are generally incorporated into the child's usual foods. For children who do not have access to adequate micronutrients and are also energy-deficient, a broader focus on improving the energy and micronutrient content of the diet, with supplements where necessary, may be more appropriate than micronutrient powders. Neumann *et al.* (2003) write that food-based approaches offer more protection than pharmaceutical approaches such as micronutrient powders because food is more locally available, because protein–energy malnutrition often coexists with micronutrient deficiencies and because food includes multiple micronutrients and thus may address deficiencies more effectively than single micronutrients or combinations of micronutrients.

In an evaluation of the impact of such powders, De-Regil *et al.* (2011) reviewed results from eight trials in developing countries and found that home use of multiple micronutrient powders containing at least iron, vitamin A and zinc reduces anaemia and iron deficiency among children aged 6–23 months. Evaluations of the long-term impact of a food supplement provided to Guatemalan children in the 1960s and 1970s showed that boys who received a more nutritious supplement earned higher hourly wages as men than did boys who did not (Hoddinott *et al.*, 2008). Girls who received the more nutritious supplement grew up to have children with higher birth weights and better anthropometric measures of nutritional status than girls who did not (Berhman *et al.*, 2009).

Based on a review of complementary feeding evaluations, Dewey and Adu-Afarwuah (2008) concluded that a combination of distribution of complementary foods and nutrition education achieves better growth outcomes than education-only projects, yet education-only participants had better growth outcomes than those in the control group. As noted above, distributing the right kinds of complementary foods (or weaning foods for children transitioning away from breastfeeding) is important.

School-aged children

School-feeding programmes typically have multiple objectives, including school enrolment and educational attainment, especially by girls, as well as nutritional outcomes. Evidence for the cost-effectiveness of school-feeding across these objectives is limited (Margolies and Hoddinott, 2012). Some researchers argue that school-feeding programmes are more effective in achieving educational goals than in improving broader measures of children's nutritional status (Afridi, 2011). Other researchers suggest that other programmes, such as conditional cash-transfers, are more effective even in terms of non-nutritional goals such as increased enrolment (Coady and Parker, 2004).

Nutrition evaluations show that school-feeding programmes can affect child nutritional status, particularly when they incorporate certain types of food. For example, including biofortified orange-fleshed sweet potato, which is high in beta-carotene, into a South African school-feeding programme raised levels of vitamin A (van Jaarsveld *et al.*, 2005). In a controlled primary school-feeding study in Kenya, children receiving milk and/or meat supplements with mid-morning snacks had higher intakes of several nutrients, including vitamins A and B_{12}, calcium, iron or zinc, and greater dietary energy (Murphy *et al.*, 2003; Neumann *et al.*, 2003). Fortifying rice served in school lunches in India led to statistically significant declines in iron-deficiency anaemia, from 30 percent to 15 percent for the treatment group, while anaemia remained essentially unchanged for the control group (Moretti *et al.*, 2006).[23]

Despite the mixed evidence regarding the cost-effectiveness of school-feeding

[23] Importantly, unlike other foods, in which iron is detectable and therefore inhibits consumption, rice fortified with iron seems to be indistinguishable from non-fortified rice (Moretti *et al.*, 2006).

programmes in achieving nutritional objectives, they remain politically popular, perhaps because they address multiple socially desirable goals such as female school attendance. In some cases, school-feeding programmes use a holistic approach to improving nutrition by not only providing food but also using school gardens, including nutrition in the curricula and other related activities. Such integrated programmes tend to be more effective and may also help to establish good lifelong eating and exercise habits, especially when combined with broader nutrition education programmes (see below).

Food assistance programmes for adults with special nutritional needs

Some food assistance programmes target vulnerable adults who need external support, such as those who are unlikely to be economically independent and thus unable to meet their basic needs. Elderly people, households with HIV-positive members, disabled people and others facing chronic illnesses are likely to fall in this category. For these people, food assistance programmes can be a major source of reliable support. External assistance can also alleviate the demands they make on local community reserves to meet needs in times of crisis.

Food assistance can provide important support to the health of HIV-positive individuals and may delay or prevent the progression of the virus. International guidance on the intersection of nutrition, food security and HIV/AIDS does exist, but work remains to be done to understand fully which foods can best support the health and nutrition of persons living with HIV/AIDS (World Bank, 2007b; Ivers *et al.*, 2009).

The evidence base on the cost-effectiveness of food assistance programmes targeting adults with special needs also needs to be strengthened. Most such interventions are motivated on humanitarian grounds, which may help explain the paucity of evidence.

Food security and nutrition interventions in protracted crises

The nutritional needs of people in countries suffering from protracted crises are a particular concern. In these countries, the proportion of people undernourished is almost three times as high as in other developing countries. The levels of stunting and the mortality rate of children under five years of age are also much worse (FAO and WFP, 2010).

These countries often need significant assistance because, in most cases, their population is facing the collapse of livelihood systems and the country has insufficient institutional capabilities to deal with crises. Most of the aid to countries in protracted crisis is humanitarian, notably food aid, while much less is development assistance (Afghanistan and Iraq are exceptions). Relatively small amounts of aid flow to agriculture and education, two sectors of particular importance for food security and nutrition. For example, only 3.1 percent of overseas development assistance received by countries in protracted crisis in the period 2005–08 was dedicated to agriculture (FAO and WFP, 2010).

The nature of the aid is also a reflection that, in the short term, immediate nutritional needs must be met. Food-assistance safety nets, such as food or cash transfers, mother and child nutrition programmes and school meal programmes, are life-saving interventions that also help preserve human capital in these countries.

In the longer term, however, programmes need to support livelihoods and build the livelihood resilience of households so they can avoid divesting themselves of their current assets and, instead, build the foundation of long-term food and nutrition security – including being able to prepare for and deal with future risks (FAO and WFP, 2010).

Nutrition-specific food price subsidies and taxes

Beyond the general food subsidies that have been used to protect food security and to increase the consumption of staple foods, food price interventions can be used more systematically to promote nutritious diets. The economic costs to society imposed by malnutrition – in terms of lost productivity and health care costs – may justify government intervention in markets through nutrition-specific food price subsidies and taxes to shape consumption patterns and diets.

As discussed above, staple foods such as rice and wheat have long been subsidized in many countries to address problems of food insecurity. Less commonly, price subsidies have been used to encourage the consumption of more diverse foods such as fruits and vegetables. Taxes can also be used to discourage the consumption of foods and beverages that are deemed less nutritious. Proposals for such taxes are increasingly common and they have been tried in several places (Capacci *et al.*, 2012; Eyles *et al.*, 2012; Mozaffarian *et al.*, 2012).

Assessments of the nutritional impacts of nutrition-specific food subsidies and taxes vary, but are generally consistent with economic theory; that is, people tend to consume more of foods that are subsidized and less of foods that are taxed. Such policies may have unintended effects, however, because a price change for one item can affect demand for that good as well as for goods that substitute for it (e.g. a tax on sugar-sweetened beverages may increase demand for beer) or that complement it (e.g. a tax on salt may reduce consumption of vegetables). Some of these cross-price effects may not lead to better nutritional choices. Because poor consumers are more responsive to price changes than affluent consumers, tax and subsidy policies may have disproportional impacts on different population groups. Moreover, many foods contain a combination of nutrients that may be beneficial or harmful depending on the amount consumed and the nutritional status of the consumer. These and other factors pose challenges to the effective use of nutrition-specific taxes and subsidies to improve dietary choices and nutritional outcomes.

Consumer food price subsidies

Consumer price subsidies have long been used to lower consumer prices of staple foods in an effort to increase consumption of those staples by the general population or by targeted groups within the larger population. Examples include subsidies on cereals in China and India (Shimokawa, 2010; Sharma, 2012).

In response to the rice price crisis of 2007 and 2008, several Asian countries used consumer price subsidies and reductions in value-added taxes (along with other types of market intervention) to moderate domestic prices of staple foods (ESCAP, 2009). Caution must be exercised in designing such subsidies, because they can be expensive and difficult to remove. In some cases, particularly when not effectively targeted, they can lead to increased prevalence of overweight and obesity when they encourage overconsumption of energy-rich, less-nutritious foods. In Egypt, subsidies on bread, wheat flour, sugar and cooking oil are considered by some to have led to excessive energy intake and to be partly responsible for the country's high prevalence of overweight and obesity (Asfaw, 2007).

The use of subsidies to encourage the consumption of more nutritious foods, including fruits and vegetables, is a recent phenomenon (Mozafarrian *et al.*, 2012; Capacci *et al.*, 2012). Several studies have shown that lowering the price of low-fat foods available in vending machines is associated with increased consumption of those foods. Some interventions have indicated that even after removing subsidies from the healthier food products, participants continued to consume relatively larger amounts than previously. This suggests that changes in preference for more healthy foods may be sustainable once new habits are established (Mozaffarian *et al.*, 2012).

Taxes on consumer food prices

As noted earlier, reductions in value-added taxes on staple foods have been used to increase food consumption to a level that satisfies energy requirements. However, food taxes to improve nutrition are normally considered in terms of how increased taxes can be used to address problems of overweight and obesity by discouraging the consumption of foods thought to be less nutritious (such as foods and beverages that are high in sugar or fat content).

Many studies of the impact of food taxes are based on simulation exercises. A recent systematic review of 32 simulation studies in OECD countries found that taxes on soft drinks and foods high in saturated fats could reduce consumption and improve health outcomes (Eyles *et al.*, 2012). A simulation exercise in the United States of America showed that among adolescents a 10 percent increase in the price of a fast-food meal was associated with a 3 percent higher probability of consuming fruits and vegetables and a 6 percent lower probability of being overweight (Powell *et al.*, 2007). A simulation study from the United Kingdom showed that taxing less-healthy foods by 17.5 percent could avert as many as 2 900 deaths a year due to cardiovascular disease and cancer, and that using the revenues from these taxes to subsidize fruits and vegetables could avert an additional 6 400 such deaths (Nnoaham *et al.*, 2009).

Studies of existing food tax policies in Europe and Northern America generally find that tax rates are too low to have a noticeable impact on consumption patterns (Mozaffarian, 2012; Capacci *et al.*, 2012; Mazzocchi, Shankar and Traill, 2012; Eyles *et al.*, 2012). Such taxes are, however, effective in raising government revenue that may be used to cover the health costs associated with overweight and obesity or to promote consumption of more nutritious foods. A simulation study in the United States of America showed that a 1 percent value-added tax on salty snacks would not reduce sales greatly, but it would generate up to US$100 million in annual revenues, which could be used for nutrition programmes (Kuchler, Tegene and Harris, 2004).

Sugar-sweetened beverage consumption by young people has emerged in recent years as a particular focus of public policy. In the United States of America, 33 states levy taxes of around 5 percent on the sale of such drinks. Simulation studies suggest that taxes of 15–20 percent would be required to have an appreciable effect on consumption (Brownell *et al.*, 2009). A 20 percent tax on all sugar-sweetened beverages could reduce consumption by only about 7 kcal per person per day, while a 40 percent tax could reduce consumption by about 12 kcal per day (Finkelstein *et al.*, 2010). Although small, these changes could contribute to weight losses of 0.3–0.6 kg per person per year and generate up to US$2.5 billion in tax revenue (Finkelstein *et al.*, 2010).

These simulations illustrate the complexity involved in designing interventions that improve nutritional outcomes for everyone. Taxing pork in China, for example, could reduce consumption of excess energy and saturated fats by higher-income consumers who are at risk of overweight and obesity, while at the same time cause an undesired decline in protein consumption by the poor (Guo *et al.*, 1999). Thus, taxes on some energy-dense foods could help address overweight and obesity but exacerbate problems of undernutrition and micronutrient deficiencies for members of poor households.

Taxing a single food or food ingredient may not lead to an overall improvement in diets because people could increase consumption of other similarly unhealthy items. Real-world experience from Denmark, France, Hungary, the United States of America and elsewhere suggests that such taxes are difficult to implement and politically unpopular. Denmark, for example, instituted a tax on fatty foods in 2011, including dairy products, meat and high-fat processed foods, but repealed it one year later. The tax was unpopular because it applied to a wide variety of foods, including traditional local delicacies such as cheeses, and it was commonly circumvented by shoppers who could easily shop in neighbouring countries (Strom, 2012).

Nutrition education

Education, including both general education and nutrition-specific education, are effective means of improving nutrition (Webb and Block, 2004; World Bank, 2007b; Headey, 2011). Maternal education – including education that improves the mother's care for herself as well as the care and feeding behaviours she provides for her family – is particularly important. Education that occurs in conjunction with other interventions to improve access to diverse, nutritious foods can be particularly effective, as noted in the discussion of food assistance programmes above.

Nutrition education is often defined broadly as holistic programmes that include an ensemble of information-related interventions aimed at increasing consumers' knowledge of what constitutes good nutrition. The ultimate goal is a change in behaviour so that individuals choose more nutritious diets and healthier lifestyles. Such programmes may include elements of nutrition training, public information campaigns and regulation of advertising and labelling, as well as improvements to the local food environment.

Nutrition training

Nutrition training provided to mothers can have a positive effect on child growth and micronutrient deficiencies, primarily through improving breastfeeding practices and complementary feeding during the weaning of young children (Bhutta *et al.*, 2008; Horton, Alderman and Rivera, 2008). Impacts are heightened when the interventions are culturally sensitive, easily accessible and based on local products (Shi and Zhang, 2011). A recent global review of 17 studies conducted in low- and middle-income countries confirmed that provision of nutritional counselling to mothers along with nutritious complementary foods can lead to significant gains in the weight and height of children aged 6-24 months (Imdad, Yakoob and Bhutta, 2011). Nutrition training can also guide households in how to consume adequate amounts of energy and micronutrients through dietary diversification. The content of such education programmes can provide knowledge and practical skills for acquiring and preparing nutritious, balanced diets.

The most effective way to ensure that education results in actual changes in behaviour is to ensure a supportive environment, because it is difficult for households to use new knowledge if other factors discourage its use (McNulty, 2013). For example, Sherman and Muehlhoff (2007) found that nutrition education is more effective when accompanied by improvements to sanitation.

Other factors, such as women's empowerment, better access to health services, or the accompanying provision of complementary foods, can also help create a supportive environment and improve nutritional outcomes. Interventions should take care to address these issues, by not only providing information about the importance of dietary diversity, for example, but suggesting specific ways to achieve it within the household budget. Peru's programme, "La Mejor Compra", is one such example (INCAP, 2013).

Notwithstanding the need for a supportive food environment, evidence shows that nutrition education can have a positive impact on dietary choices even when households face constraints. When confronted with sharp increases in staple food prices, for example, Indonesian households that were knowledgeable about nutrition attempted to protect their consumption of micronutrient-rich foods relatively more than those without such knowledge (Block, 2003).

In contrast, as mentioned in Chapter 3, households lacking such knowledge tend to reduce consumption of micronutrient-rich foods when faced with price shocks. Other factors being equal, mothers who had practical nutritional knowledge and skills allocated a larger share of their food budget to micronutrient-rich foods. Significantly, this difference was even larger at lower-income levels. This suggests that knowledge about the importance of foods rich in micronutrients can increase demand for them.

Nutrition education in schools is likewise effective in addressing problems of overweight and obesity and associated non-communicable diseases, especially when combined with efforts to improve the diversity and nutritional quality of foods available. In 2011, WHO and other international organizations launched the Nutrition-Friendly Schools Initiative, which provides a framework for implementing integrated intervention programmes to improve the health and nutritional status of school-age children and adolescents and uses the school as the programme setting (including nurseries and kindergartens). This initiative brings together parents, the local community and health services to promote children's health and nutritional well-being (WHO, 2011b). It encourages pairing nutrition training with increased availability of healthier foods and restrictions on less-healthy foods and beverages in schools in order to have the greatest impact.

A review of 19 evaluations of school-based interventions found that nutrition training in schools was effective in addressing overweight and obesity, particularly when combined with efforts to increase physical activity (Mozaffarian *et al.*, 2012). Evaluations of various school-based nutrition education programmes to address overweight and obesity in Italy and Portugal found positive effects on consumption and health (Capacci *et al.*, 2012).

Comprehensive nutrition and health interventions in the workplace that include training components can also be effective (Mozaffarian *et al.*, 2012; Hawkes, 2013). WHO's Global Strategy on Diet, Physical Activity and Health and the 2011 Political Declaration of the UN High Level Meeting on the Prevention and Control of Non-communicable Diseases both support such workplace-based interventions (WHO, 2004: United Nations, 2011a).

Nutrition programmes in the workplace obviously need to involve private-sector employers, and some efforts are already being made. Along these lines, the World Economic Forum, has, for example, created a Workplace Wellness Alliance, a consortium of companies committed to improving health through workplace-based initiatives (World Economic Forum, 2012). Nestlé has implemented a nutrition education programme targeted at its more than 300 000 employees, which aims to improve their knowledge of nutrition so they can make better decisions for themselves and also improve product design (Hawkes, 2013).

Nutrition training can also be delivered in community centres and other locations. The Expanded Food and Nutrition Education Program in the United States of America is a large community-based programme sponsored by the government. Targeting low-income adults, its objective is to improve their nutritional knowledge and their ability to prepare healthy meals for their families. Programme activities are delivered in locations such as health clinics, children's centres, family resource centres, job clubs, and in the home. Recent evaluations indicate that participants are more likely to follow national food-based dietary guidelines, pay attention to nutrition labels, increase their consumption of fruits and vegetables and improve their meal planning (USDA, 2009).

Public information campaigns

Public information campaigns also play an important role in addressing malnutrition by improving households' understanding of what constitutes a nutritious diet. These campaigns have been implemented by governments and the private sector and through public–private partnerships. Such campaigns are also known as "social marketing" as they use commercial marketing methods to achieve the social good. Although comparatively inexpensive, the sustainability of public information campaigns is often tenuous, because they may rely solely on public funds, with support depending on political trends, or on private companies, which generally must justify the use of such "public" campaigns in terms of private gains.

One example of a joint public–private effort is the United Kingdom's Change4Life campaign. This aims to raise awareness, through use of the media, about the health risks associated with overweight and obesity and the importance of nutritious diets and of physical activity for good health. The programme consists of four phases: awareness-raising; assessment of the diets and physical activity levels of children; distribution of customized "family information packs" and distribution of additional information to lower-income families (Croker, Lucas and Wardle, 2012).

National food-based dietary guidelines are widely used as part of broad public information campaigns. They communicate in simple terms what constitutes an adequate and nutritious diet, thereby simplifying technical information developed by nutritionists in a way that is intelligible to the general public. They typically include a food guide, often in graphic form, such as the Chinese pagoda, the Thai nutrition flag or the United States food pyramid, which provides daily recommended intakes for different types of food. Campaigns on specific issues are also frequently used; examples include the "no sugar kid's network" in Thailand, as well as "breastfeeding week" and "micronutrient day" in Viet Nam (WHO, 2011c).

FAO and WHO have been promoting the use of such guidelines since the International Conference on Nutrition in 1992. They have evolved to include not only nutrition concerns but also food safety and recommendations concerning physical activity (Hawkes, 2013). Important recommendations for reducing malnutrition among infants are the early initiation of breastfeeding, exclusive breastfeeding for the first six months, as well as the timely introduction of complementary foods (WHO, 2011c).

Food-based dietary guidelines are widely used, though their prevalence varies by region; Hawkes (2013) has identified at least 81 countries that have developed and implemented them (4 countries in sub-Saharan Africa, 9 in the Near East and North African region, 15 in Asia and the Pacific; 2 in Northern America; 23 in Latin America and the Caribbean; and 28 in Europe). Their impact on consumption and nutritional outcomes has not been widely studied, but some evidence indicates that they improve awareness of proper nutrition (Hawkes, 2013). Nevertheless, conceptualizing, formulating and implementing these guidelines is a complex undertaking (FAO and WHO, 2006).

The impact of broad, general information campaigns on consumer behaviour appears to be somewhat limited. Capacci *et al.* (2012) assessed ten public information campaigns throughout Europe and found increased awareness and knowledge but little impact on behaviour and nutritional outcomes. These findings are consistent with an evaluation of the Change4life programme (Croker, Lucas and Wardle, 2012), as well as earlier systematic reviews of other similar programmes (National Institute for Health and Clinical Excellence, 2007; Mazzocchi, Traill and Shogren, 2009). The apparently low effectiveness of general public information campaigns may be explained by the lengthy timeframe needed to affect nutritional outcomes (Mozaffarian *et al.*, 2012). The modest size and duration of public information campaigns compared with private-sector advertising campaigns, for example, may also limit their effectiveness (California Pan-Ethnic Health Network and Consumers Union, 2005).

Public information campaigns that have a more targeted message, focusing on promoting the consumption of certain foods such as fruits and vegetables or discouraging the consumption of specific foods such as sugar, sodium and trans-fats may have greater impact. These more targeted campaigns often include complementary activities that increase the availability and accessibility of healthier choices. Campaigns to encourage increased consumption of fruits and vegetables have been undertaken in several developing countries including, Argentina, Brazil, Chile, Mexico and South Africa as well as in high-income countries in Australasia, Europe and Northern America (Hawkes, 2013).

The United Kingdom's "5 a day" campaign promoted the consumption of five servings of fruits and vegetables through a school-based programme that combined an educational component with collaboration with suppliers to increase the availability of fruits and vegetables in school lunches. An evaluation of the campaign found a 27 percent increase in fruit and vegetable consumption after the first year (Capacci and Mazzocchi, 2011).

A similar initiative in Australia, the "Go for 2 & 5", also led to increases in household consumption of the targeted food group (Pollard *et al.*, 2008). In Chile, the "5 al dia" programme led to increased awareness of the health benefits of fruit and vegetable consumption among participants, but little change was seen in their consumption of such foods (Hawkes, 2013). As with the nutrition education programmes discussed above, public information campaigns may be more effective in combination with efforts to create a more supportive environment that helps consumers make better choices.

Regulation of advertising and labelling

Whether or not advertising by food and beverage manufacturers and retailers has contributed to the rise in overweight and obesity is a matter of growing concern and sharp debate (Harris and Graff, 2012; Keller and Schulz, 2011). Commercial advertising almost certainly influences consumers' food choices and diets – otherwise, companies would be unlikely to spend the sums they do. In light of this, 85 percent of the 73 countries surveyed in a WHO review regulated television advertising targeting children (Hawkes, 2004). At the same time, many governments and international organizations have begun to call for regulation of food and beverage advertising, especially to children (Garde, 2008; Hawkes, 2013). WHO Member States have already endorsed a *Set of recommendations on the marketing of foods and non-alcoholic beverages to children*. These provide guidance to governments on the design of policies to reduce the impact on children of the marketing of foods high in saturated fats, trans-fatty acids, free sugars and salt (WHO, 2010).

The effectiveness of advertising restrictions in influencing healthy food choices and improving nutritional outcomes is debated (Mozaffarian *et al.*, 2012; Capacci *et al.*, 2012; Hawkes, 2013). Many studies in this area are based on hypothetical rather than actual restrictions. The impacts of actual restrictions seem to depend on the precise nature of the restriction and a variety of other factors that are difficult for researchers to control. For example, studies of proposed bans on food advertising to children in the United States of America suggested they would result in potential reductions of almost 15 percent in the prevalence of overweight and obesity among children (Chou, Rashad and Grossman, 2008; Veerman *et al.*, 2009). Yet evidence from regions and countries where food advertising bans have been implemented is mixed. For example, in Quebec, Canada, all food advertising to children was banned in 1980, and the ban seems to have reduced the consumption of fast foods (Dhar and Baylis, 2011). Sweden has also banned food advertising to children, but with no measurable impact on child obesity rates (Lobstein and Frelut, 2003).

Standardized nutrition labels are a source of information for consumers, with the aim of helping them make more nutritious food choices. The Joint FAO/WHO Codex Alimentarius Commission provides guidelines to governments on the use of nutrient lists for processed and packaged foods and recommends mandatory labelling when nutritional claims are made (FAO and WHO, 2012). Most developed countries require nutrient labels on all processed and packaged foods and many are also extending this requirement to foods consumed away from home. Many developing countries are also beginning to require nutrient labels on processed and packaged foods.

Studies generally show that nutrient labels influence consumer decisions, although perhaps not strongly (Variyam, 2007; Capacci *et al.*, 2012; Mozaffarian *et al.*, 2012; Siu and Man-yi Tsoi, 1998; Colón-Ramos *et al.*, 2007). Consumers seem most likely to use the information on nutrient labels when they already have enough knowledge to understand the information and have the resources to be able to act on it. Ease of use is a determining factor in the effectiveness of labels (Signal *et al.*, 2007).

Labels can be relatively ineffective in influencing the dietary choices of the poor for a variety of reasons. Poor consumers appear to attach more importance to price than to label information (Drichoutis, Panagiotis and Nayga, 2006). Furthermore, labels are used primarily for processed and packaged products and very rarely in wet markets (where the poor in developing countries are more likely to shop, see Chapter 4). For processed foods, however, when combined with nutrition education, nutrition labels are likely to encourage better food choices, more nutritious diets and better nutritional outcomes.

In addition to influencing consumers, mandatory disclosure of information about the nutritional content of food can influence the behaviour of food processors and retailers, even encouraging the reformulation of products (Ippolito and Mathias, 1993; Golan and Unnevehr, 2008; Mozaffarian *et al.*, 2012). For example, in the United States of America, the mandatory inclusion of trans-fats on nutrition labels in 2006 quickly led major brands to substitute away from trans-fats so they could position their products as trans-fat-free (Rahkovsky, Martinez and Kuchler, 2012). This shift started even before the regulation took effect, as the media, law suits and local regulation had already brought attention to the issue. It reverberated throughout the supply chain, and agricultural producers reacted by expanding production of low-linoleic soybeans (Unnevehr and Jagmanaite, 2008). The success of this labelling policy, combined with increased consumer awareness of the negative effects of trans-fats on health, was reflected in a drop of 58 percent in observed levels of trans-fats in blood samples taken from white adults between 2000 and 2009 (CDC, 2012).

In general, then, evidence regarding the effectiveness of advertising and nutrient labelling regulations on consumer behaviour and nutritional outcomes shows that such efforts can be effective, but the results are not always as predictable and also depend on a variety of other factors. Nutrition education and information are more likely to help consumers make healthy dietary choices when other parts of the food system are equally supportive.

Improving the local food environment

The local food environment, that is, the ease with which people have access to diverse nutritious food, influences their dietary choices. Measures that can improve the local food environment include increasing the availability of supermarkets, grocery stores, farmers' markets and community gardens; changing the types of foods available in stores and schools; and reducing the availability of fast-food restaurants and convenience stores (Mozaffarian *et al.*, 2012).

Governments can exert direct leverage in schools to increase the availability of nutritious foods and limit access to less-nutritious ones. Public authorities may establish standards or otherwise control the availability of the foods and beverages they offer in school cafeterias and vending machines, for example (Hawkes, 2013). Engagement with the private sector, at least in industrialized countries, has revolved largely around sugar-sweetened beverages and offerings of food products in vending machines. Though controversial, Capacci *et al.* (2012) find some evidence of the positive impact on dietary intake of regulating school vending machines.

One of the most ambitious programmes aimed at increasing the availability of nutritious foods to schoolchildren is the EU's School Fruit Scheme, introduced in 2008. The programme supports country-level initiatives to provide fruits and vegetables to schoolchildren and by 2011 had been implemented in most EU Member States (European Commission, 2012a). Evaluations indicate that it has successfully increased fruit and vegetable consumption among youth (European Commission, 2012b). Capacci *et al.* (2012) find similar results for the impact on dietary intake of other school fruit and vegetable schemes.

As suggested above, schools can serve as important platforms through which to improve food consumption and dietary patterns. The National School Lunch Program in the United States of America, for instance, provides more than 31 million children per day with a nutritious lunch and other millions of students with after-school snacks. The programme has suffered criticisms of the quality of its meals, but its menu and nutritional standards have been updated in recent years to meet the country's current dietary guidelines. This has resulted in more fruits, vegetables and whole grains on the menu (USDA, 2012).

Mozaffarian *et al.* (2012) found that holistic school-based approaches – ones that aim to improve diet and physical activity and the food environment – are the most successful in changing child nutrition. The authors note that both school-gardening programmes and programmes providing students with fruits and vegetables as snacks can increase fruit and vegetable consumption. Jaime and Lock's (2009) review of research on changes to the school food environment supports this conclusion, noting that students improved their dietary intakes following a range of interventions, such as increased availability of fruits and vegetables at school and reduced fat content of school meals.

With regard to the workplace, Mozaffarian *et al.* (2012) similarly argue for holistic worksite wellness programmes that incorporate various measures to improve food consumption patterns, including education as well as improvements to the food environment. Few of these efforts have so far been evaluated for impact (Capacci *et al.*, 2012).

Conclusions and key messages

Consumer choices are at the nexus of nutrition and sustainability. Their choices influence consumers' own nutritional status as well as what is produced by food systems and how sustainable production and consumption patterns can be. Evidence shows that consumer choices are influenced by their access to nutritious foods, their knowledge regarding healthy diets and direct incentives and disincentives for the consumption of particular foods. Governments can influence the design of food assistance programmes to promote better nutritional outcomes. They can regulate the nutrition training, public information, advertising and labelling to which consumers are exposed and they can influence the quality of local food environments by encouraging the availability of more diverse foods. Governments can give consumers the information they need and make it easier for them to make healthy choices, but ultimately consumers must choose.

Key messages

- Nutritional outcomes ultimately depend on consumer choices. Governments play an important role in shaping the food environment and ensuring that consumers have the knowledge and information they need to make healthy choices.
- Food assistance programmes could improve nutritional outcomes by better targeting of more flexible forms of assistance. Food assistance may be more effective in achieving nutritional goals when combined with nutrition education.
- Incentives can play an important role in shaping consumer behaviour and nutritional outcomes, but they may have unintended consequences. Such policies should be based on sound evidence regarding what constitutes a healthy diet.
- Nutrition education is likely to be more effective when it consists of a set of interventions including, for example, elements of nutrition training, public information campaigns, improved food environments, and training and awareness-raising about the importance of physical activity.

6. Institutional and policy environment for nutrition

Good nutrition contributes to a healthy and productive life, but malnutrition remains a significant problem in many regions and imposes a high cost on individuals and societies. Sustainable solutions to malnutrition of all types (undernutrition, micronutrient deficiencies and overweight and obesity) must involve different sectors, but food systems and the policies and institutions that shape them are fundamental for better nutrition.

By assessing and shaping each element of the food system, policy-makers, producers, consumers and other stakeholders can create a more "nutritious" food system, in which food selections are available, accessible, diverse and nutritious. And this goal must include production and consumption patterns that are more sustainable. This aspiration is reflected in the basic principles advocated by international development institutions and inter-agency UN bodies to enhance the impacts of agricultural programmes, policies and investments on nutrition (Box 11).

The food system is an essential element of any strategy to improve nutrition, but it is part of an interconnected set of sectors and systems, including health and sanitation. This report focuses on what food systems can bring to the nutrition table. It identifies and reviews the evidence for actions that can be taken at different stages of the food system – from production to consumption – to improve nutrition. This food-based approach is often contrasted with more medical approaches that rely on supplements. Supplements are warranted in some cases, but consuming a diet adequate in energy and micronutrients is usually sufficient and provides the benefits from the whole diverse complex of energy, nutrients and fibre present in the diet.

The complex causes of nutrition and the wide range of participants influencing food systems mean that a multistakeholder and multisectoral approach will be most effective.[24] Implicitly, this means understanding the relationships among the actors, how they tie together and how they influence one another. Considering the entire food system in addressing nutrition provides a framework in which to determine, design and implement food-based interventions to improve nutrition. Food systems are changing rapidly, but how they evolve can be influenced by policy decisions.

Building a common vision

Considerable effort and large sums of money have been devoted to addressing malnutrition worldwide. Progress has been made: in some countries malnutrition has been markedly reduced over recent decades. But progress has been uneven and there is a pressing need to harness the opportunities within the food system to enhance nutrition. Experience in several countries that have implemented nutrition programmes shows that it is imperative to build a common vision of nutrition. At the international level, the Scaling Up Nutrition (SUN) movement, the Right to Food principles and other initiatives, such as the UN REACH (Renewed Efforts Against Child Hunger and undernutrition) partnership, work towards providing necessary frameworks and support (Box 12). At the same time external input can be a catalyst for national action.

A common vision can be established by setting the nutrition strategy in terms of national poverty reduction and sustainable consumption. For example, in Peru, civil society and other stakeholders, coming together in the Child Nutrition Initiative, worked towards including nutrition goals in

[24] See World Bank (2013) for guidance on mainstreaming nutrition interventions into multisectoral action, with a focus on agriculture, social protection and health.

BOX 11
Guiding principles for improving nutrition through agriculture

A FAO systematic review of recently published guidance on agriculture programming for nutrition (Herforth, 2013) identified an emerging consensus around the following recommendations:

Planning for nutrition

1. **Incorporate explicit nutrition objectives** in agricultural policy and programme design.
2. **Assess the context** and causes of malnutrition at the local level, to maximize effectiveness and reduce negative side effects.
3. **Do no harm.** Identify potential harms, develop a mitigation plan, and set in place a well-functioning monitoring system.
4. **Measure nutritional impact through programme monitoring and evaluation.**
5. Maximize opportunities through **multisectoral coordination.**
6. **Maximize impact of household income** on nutrition, such as through increasing women's income.
7. **Increase equitable access to productive resources.**
8. **Target the most vulnerable.**

Taking action

All approaches should:

9. **Empower women,** the primary caretakers in households, through: income; access to extension services and information; avoiding harm to their ability to care for children; labour and time-saving technologies; and support for rights to land, education and employment.
10. **Incorporate nutrition education** to improve consumption and nutrition effects of interventions. Employ agricultural extension agents to communicate on nutrition as feasible.
11. **Manage natural resources** for improved productivity, resilience to shocks, adaptation to climate change, and increased equitable access to resources through soil, water and biodiversity conservation.

These can be combined with approaches to:

12. **Diversify production and livelihoods** for improved food access and dietary diversification, natural resource management, risk reduction and improved income.
13. **Increase production of nutritious foods,** particularly locally adapted varieties rich in micronutrients and protein, chosen based on local nutrition issues and available solutions.
14. **Reduce post-harvest losses and improve processing.**
15. **Increase market access and opportunities,** especially for smallholders.
16. **Reduce seasonality of food insecurity** through improved storage and preservation and other approaches.

Creating a supportive environment

17. **Improve policy coherence** supportive to nutrition, including food price policies, subsidies, trade policies and pro-poor policies.
18. **Improve good governance for nutrition,** by drawing up a national nutrition strategy and action plan, allocating adequate budgetary resources and implementing nutrition surveillance.
19. **Build capacity** in ministries at national, district and local levels.
20. **Communicate and continue to advocate for nutrition.**

BOX 12
Nutrition governance at the international level

The causes of malnutrition are manifold and a number of different sectors, ranging from agriculture, health, education, social affairs, economic development and trade, among others, are involved. Nevertheless, while nutrition is everybody's business, it lacks an institutional home. A functioning international nutrition governance structure is essential to provide leadership and coordination and help surmount the challenges posed by the multisectoral nature of the fight to eliminate malnutrition.

Globally, attention to nutrition has never been higher and the renewed interest in nutrition is matched by an increased willingness to work together. In some cases, this has given rise to new multisectoral collaboration platforms (e.g. SUN and REACH). Similarly, it has reinforced the importance of existing joint efforts (e.g. the UN Standing Committee on Nutrition [UNSCN], Emergency Nutrition Cluster). These mechanisms can help foster collaboration among UN and other international agencies that have mandates linked directly or indirectly to food security and nutritional outcomes. They also facilitate multisectoral and multistakeholder dialogue and collaboration. However, an understanding of their distinctions and complementarities is important in order to engage with and leverage them effectively.

The **UN Standing Committee on Nutrition** (UNSCN) aligns and coordinates technical and policy guidance and programming among the UN agencies working on nutrition. It provides global strategic leadership, advocacy, guidance and knowledge exchange on nutrition across the UN system and for non-UN planners.

Scaling-Up Nutrition (SUN) is a country-owned movement, established in 2010, that has helped elevate nutrition on the policy agenda at international and national levels. It includes governments, UN agencies, research organizations, civil society organizations, NGOs, the private sector and international development agencies and partners. The SUN Framework primarily focuses on scaling up interventions that target conception through the first two years of life (Bezanson and Isenman, 2010). A SUN roadmap has been devised, providing practical guidelines for joint action to be adopted on a country-by-country basis. Over 100 organizations and 28 countries have joined SUN.

The **REACH** (Renewed Efforts Against Child Hunger and undernutrition) partnership was established by FAO, the United Nations Children's Fund (UNICEF), the World Food Programme (WFP) and WHO to facilitate, support and coordinate action on nutrition among stakeholders at country level. It promotes a holistic approach to tackling undernutrition in the context of the Millennium Development Goal (MDG) 1, with a view to helping governments plan, prioritize and manage inter-sectoral nutrition activities among multiple stakeholders.

The relationships among UNSCN, REACH and SUN are mutually supportive. UNSCN works toward strategic coherence in policy and programming for the UN. REACH harnesses the work of these agencies to support country governments in combating malnutrition, particularly in fulfilling their commitments in the fight against malnutrition to SUN and other bodies. As a stakeholder within SUN, the UNSCN can serve as the voice of the UN in dealing with nutrition matters.

The Global Cluster Coordination Group brings together agencies and organizations from inside and outside the UN. The goal is to improve effectiveness of humanitarian response and strengthened partnership among UN and non-UN actors. UNICEF leads the global **Nutrition Cluster**, WHO the global **Health Cluster** and FAO/WFP jointly lead the **Global Food Security Cluster**, whereas the leads of the respective country-level clusters

(CONT.)

BOX 12 *(CONT.)*

are determined according to capacity on the ground. Nevertheless, each cluster provides concrete tools and support for coordination, emergency preparedness, assessment, monitoring and capacity development.

In the spirit of UN Reform, a few joint programming schemes have been created to foster increased harmonization and efficiency within the UN system. Among these, experiences from the UN Joint Programmes and the joint programmes for the thematic window on Children, Nutrition and Food Security of the MDG Fund have shown that nutrition is an effective entry point to joint planning. The UN Development Assistance Framework guides integration of efforts by UN agencies.

The **Alliance Against Hunger and Malnutrition** (AAHM) is a global initiative that links UN agencies, governments, civil society organizations and NGOs in a coalition for advocacy and action. It provides a space where governments and civil society organizations can find their similarities and build working relationships. The potential contribution of these country-led partnerships has been recognized by global mechanisms such as the High Level Task Force on the Global Food Security Crisis and the Committee on World Food Security.

Numerous international initiatives are focused on addressing overweight and obesity as well as relevant non-communicable diseases. These include the WHO Global Strategy on Diet, Physical Activity and Health adopted by the World Health Assembly in 2004, as well as the WHO 2008–2013 Action Plan for implementing the strategy. Another key effort is the Political Declaration of the High-level Meeting of the General Assembly on the Prevention and Control of Non-communicable Diseases, which was passed by the General Assembly of the United Nations in 2011.

the poverty reduction strategy (IDS, 2012). In Brazil, the Campaign Against Hunger and the subsequent *Fome Zero* programme were set within a poverty and hunger reduction strategy, thus making the programme not only a health sector issue. In Senegal, nutrition was included as a development priority in the national poverty reduction strategy.

Experience in countries with successful nutrition strategies, such as Brazil, Peru and Senegal, shows that strong and committed political leadership is essential for success (Acosta and Fanzo, 2012; Garrett and Natalicchio, 2011). Strong political leadership, as seen in Brazil, is essential for building coalitions and strong policy commitment. This is so also because nutrition does not usually have an institutional home, such as a ministry of nutrition.

It is inevitable that policy-makers and other actors will have different, sometimes conflicting, views about nutrition problems. In part, this is because malnutrition is often invisible; the malnourished are often without voice; and because interventions need to be cross-sectoral. A key step towards creating a common vision is to bring the various sectors and stakeholders together. For example, in Uganda this process started with stakeholder fora organized by the health sector (Namugumya, 2012). A nutrition advocacy technical working group was also formed for Uganda, comprising health and agriculture but also education, gender, population and agencies responsible for statistics, civil society, the media and academia.

Raising the profile of malnutrition outcomes and policy must follow from the common vision. Effective advocacy is needed for this. In India, the Right to Food Campaign has been highly effective, also because it has been able to develop a strong narrative on the severity of undernutrition, making nutrition visible and placing it on the policy agenda. The Campaign works closely with the National Advisory Council and the Commissioners of the Supreme Court to maintain pressure for policy action and results. Accountability is needed to ensure that nutrition remains visible and that plans turn into actions and results. Advocacy and accountability will be effective only when civil society is fully involved and engaged in the political process at all levels. Benson (2008) and Namugumya (2012) emphasize the importance of actively cultivating policy champions within government institutions, who become the visible leaders who will advocate making health and nutrition a priority of government and government institutions.

Better data for better policy-making

Effective policy-making, accountability and advocacy depend on a correct assessment of the nutrition situation. This report showed that in many countries there is a lack of basic data and indicators with which to evaluate and monitor the nutrition landscape. This is also a reflection of the limited research carried out on the linkages between the food system and nutrition, research that is needed to design efficient data collection and help develop cost-effective indicators.

The absence of adequate data proved a challenge in Colombia when preparing the Food and Nutrition Improvement Plan of Antioquia (Garrett and Natalicchio, 2011). In Ethiopia, a 2005 survey showed that malnutrition was highest in the regions with highest agricultural productivity. This counter-intuitive situation might not have been recognized without such survey data. Accurate and timely nutrition data also contribute to the effectiveness of advocacy initiatives (IDS, 2012). Collecting outcome data at regular intervals is important for building consensus, coordination and allocation of funds. As such, the demand for information must also be managed across sectors. Effective monitoring is an important part of nutrition governance.

Effective coordination is essential

Because malnutrition has multiple causes – poor diets, unclean water, poor sanitation, illness and poor child care – multisectoral interventions are therefore required and these need to be coordinated. The experience of UN Joint Programmes, in particular the programme area "Children, Food Security and Nutrition" of the MDG Achievement Fund, shows the importance of coordination among all involved stakeholders, particularly local governments and civil society (MDG Achievement Fund, 2013).

Effective horizontal coordination is one of the key features of the success of *Fome Zero* and other, albeit less ambitious, programmes. In Brazil, formulation, adoption and implementation of nutrition policies is coordinated by the National System of Food Security and Nutrition (SISAN). This system consists of 17 ministries and is led by the President. Also in Brazil, the Congress has contributed to intersectoral collaboration through legitimizing policy initiatives and facilitating communication among different stakeholders such as ministries, state and municipal governments and civil society (Acosta, 2011a). Civil society has also played an important part through the National Council on Food Security (Conselho Nacional de Segurança Alimentar e Nutricional – CONSEA) which consists of two-thirds civil society members and one-third government representatives. CONSEA provides support, monitoring and policy advice in the formulation of food and nutrition policies and programmes.

In Peru, success in reducing malnutrition was in part due to economic growth, but more due to improved national coordination structures and mechanisms, more public and private spending on nutrition programmes and the alignment of social programmes with the national nutrition strategy (Acosta, 2011b). An important role in fostering dialogue and coordination was played by the Roundtable for Poverty Reduction (Mesa de Concertación para la Lucha Contra la Pobreza – MCLCP). Since the 1980s, there have been many attempts to establish similar bodies in Latin America and the Caribbean but many had a limited impact because of mixed coordination and dialogue functions, the lack of adequate funding and resources and a lack of political will. The examples of CONSEA and MCLCP demonstrate which factors facilitate the successful implementation of mechanisms and bodies that improve the governance of food and nutrition security. There are differences, but the main lessons are common to both:

- The process must be country-driven.
- Separate bodies are needed for internal government coordination and for dialogue on policies, participation and coordination of stakeholders' efforts.

- Institutional arrangements must have adequate resources.
- Decentralized bodies must be established to enable these mechanisms to work at national and subnational levels.

The importance of intersectoral coordination is also highlighted by the experience of Bangladesh, where nutrition policy has evolved over a lengthy period. For a number of reasons, multisectoral coordination has been weak and although donors play an important role, they seem to focus on accountability at the programme level rather than on coordination across sectors (Taylor, 2012a). Donor support has clearly been crucial but has not provided the framework or incentives for cross-sectoral cooperation and programming.

In India, malnutrition has become an issue of importance to policy-makers through a combination of judicial activism, the Commissioners of the Supreme Court, a Right to Food Campaign and media attention. In 2001, a series of court orders gave legal entitlements to government interventions on malnutrition. The Right to Food Campaign, which grew out of the court case, was a key factor in putting malnutrition on the policy agenda. Despite these developments, there appears to be relatively little intersectoral coordination between state and non-state agencies and even across ministries. A recent analysis found that there are no coordinating bodies, integrated work plans or joint budget lines to deal with malnutrition (Mohmand, 2012).

In many countries, significant challenges have hampered coordination efforts thus far. Lack of funding and qualified nutritionists and the inability to convene high-level actors have been identified as key constraints (Taylor, 2012b). Coordination can be enhanced through multisectoral policy reviews and impact assessments. For example, an impact assessment for agricultural projects could include health and nutrition outcome indicators. At the same time, incentives that encourage cross-sectoral collaboration are needed. Garrett and Natalicchio (2011) note that institutional links that are built on joint incentives – both financial and success sharing – is essential for coordination to be effective.

In Africa, planning and coordination are facilitated by the New Partnership for Africa's Development (NEPAD). Efforts are now being made to integrate nutrition into the National Agricultural and Food Security Investment Plans, established under the Comprehensive Africa Agriculture Development Programme (CAADP).

Effective vertical coordination is also needed. A highly centralized decision-making process, for financial planning and programme design, leads to lack of coordination with local communities and at the local level itself. Service delivery is more effective at the community level, that is, when decentralized. Multisectoral collaboration is also easier at the subnational level. Vertical coordination is therefore very important but is only effective when there is capacity to deliver. Building incentives for collaboration among central, state and local government is essential to achieve this goal.

The incentives from greater intersectoral cooperation and improved vertical cooperation come in part through the particular funding modalities. For example, *Bolsa Família*, in Brazil, tied payments to poorer families to school attendance and regular health checks, so creating an incentive for coordination between the Health and Education Ministries. Similarly, the school lunch programme was tied to food purchases from local producers. The Brazilian government also provided additional support to poorer municipalities to implement the *Bolsa Família* programme (Acosta, 2011a). In general, transparency in budget allocation is a critical factor for continued intersectoral collaboration.

Introduction of new seed types or food products requires legislation and regulation that deal with, for example, environmental and health issues. Here again, cross-sectoral collaboration plays an important role. For example, in Burkina Faso and Mali the Ministries of the Environment play a leading role in biosafety regulation, but the Ministry of Health also is an important actor, as is the Ministry of Agriculture. At the same time, farmer organizations, rural women's organizations, consumer organizations, NGOs and the food industry are directly involved and each will try to influence the process in its interest (Birner *et al.*, 2007). Legislation and regulation are also relevant to the challenge of supply chain governance, which grows more complex with the food system transformation.

Agencies must have the capacity to coordinate, plan, implement, monitor and evaluate. In Zambia, increasing the number of qualified nutritionists in the main coordinating body may improve coordination (Taylor, 2012b). Staff training in nutrition is important also to help develop a common language amongst actors in different sectors. In Senegal, qualified NGOs and training allowed the Nutrition Enhancement Program to work well at the local level (Garrett and Natalicchio, 2011).

A great many actors and institutions must work together across sectors to more effectively reduce undernutrition, micronutrient deficiencies and overweight and obesity. Good governance, that is, providing leadership, coordinating effectively and fostering collaboration among the many stakeholders, is a first priority.

Key messages of the report

The State of Food and Agriculture 2013: Food systems for better nutrition offers the following key messages:

- **Malnutrition in all its forms imposes unacceptably high costs on society in human and economic terms.** The costs associated with undernutrition and micronutrient deficiencies are higher than those associated with overweight and obesity, although the latter are rising rapidly even in low- and middle-income countries.
- **Addressing malnutrition requires a multisectoral approach that includes complementary interventions in food systems, public health and education.** This approach also facilitates the pursuit of multiple objectives, including better nutrition, gender equality and environmental sustainability.
- **Within a multisectoral approach, food systems offer many opportunities for interventions leading to improved diets and better nutrition.** Some of these interventions have the primary purpose of enhancing nutrition. Other interventions in food systems, and in the general economic, social or political environment, may affect nutrition even though this is not their primary objective.
- **Agricultural production and productivity growth remain essential for better nutrition, but more can be done.** Agricultural research must continue to enhance productivity, while paying greater attention to nutrient-dense foods such as fruits, vegetables, legumes and animal products and to more sustainable production systems. Production interventions are more effective when they are sensitive to gender roles and combined with nutrition education.
- **Both traditional and modern supply chains offer risks and opportunities for achieving better nutrition and more sustainable food systems.** Improvements in traditional supply chains can help reduce losses, lower prices and increase diversity of choice for lower-income households. The growth of modern retailing and food processing can facilitate the use of fortification to combat malnutrition, but the increased availability of highly processed, packaged goods may contribute to overweight and obesity.
- **Consumers ultimately determine what they eat and therefore what the food system produces.** But governments, international organizations, the private sector and civil society can all help consumers make healthier decisions, reduce waste and contribute to the sustainable use of resources, by providing clear, accurate information and ensuring access to diverse and nutritious foods.
- **Better governance of food systems at all levels, facilitated by high-level political support, is needed to build a common vision, to support evidence-based policies, and to promote effective coordination and collaboration through integrated, multisectoral action.**

STATISTICAL ANNEX

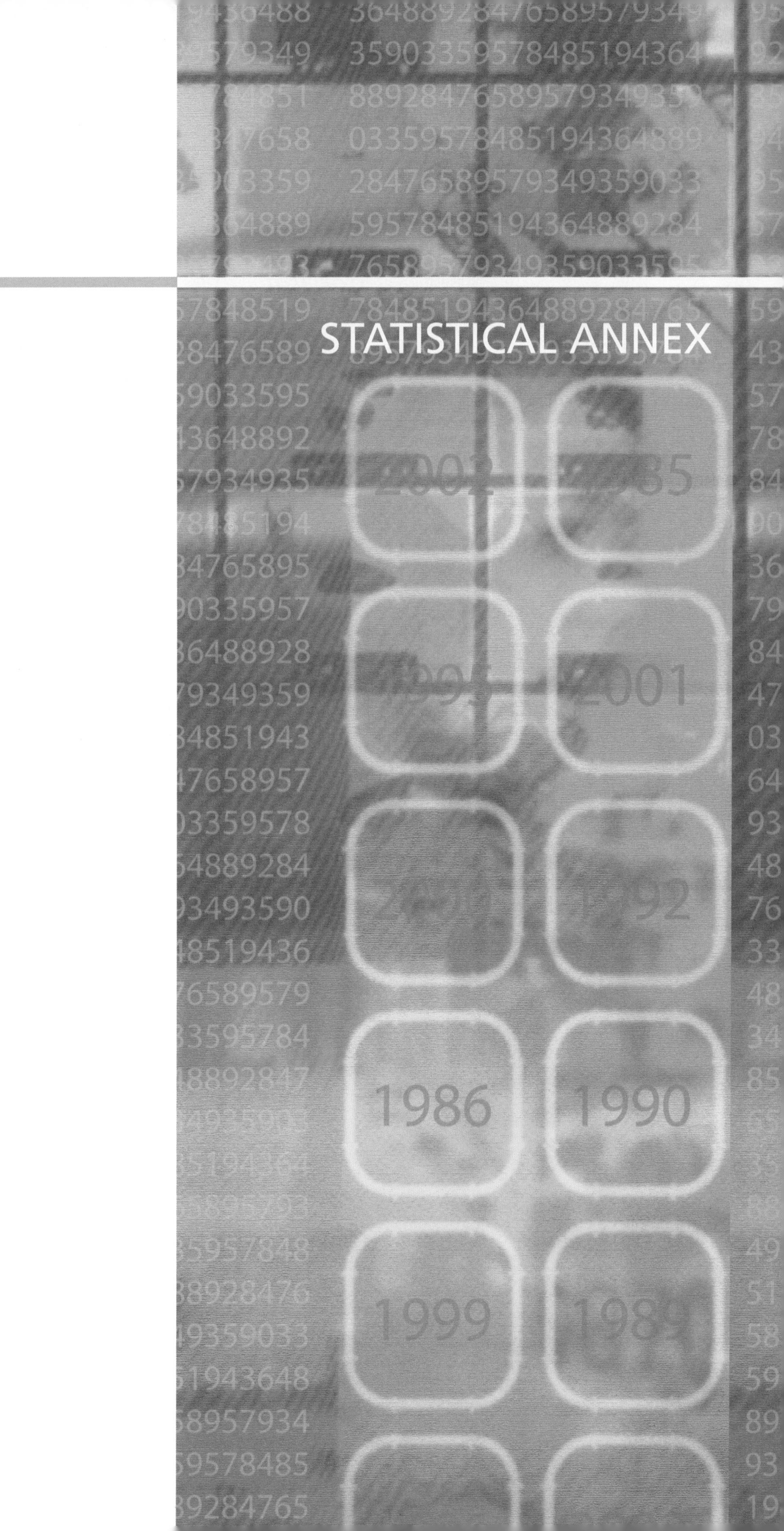

Notes for the annex table

Key

The following conventions are used in the table:

..	= data not available
0 or 0.0	= nil or negligible
blank cell	= not applicable

Numbers presented in the annex table may differ from the original data sources because of rounding or data processing. To separate decimals from whole numbers a full point (.) is used.

Technical notes

Prevalence of stunting among children

Sources: UNICEF, WHO and the World Bank, 2012 and United Nations, 2011b. At the country level, observations are for the most recent year available. (A) indicates that regional aggregates (for both Central and Southern Asia) are FAO estimates using the data presented and age-specific population weights (United Nations, 2011b). All other regional aggregates are modelled estimates for the year 2010 as presented in UNICEF, WHO and World Bank (2012).

Stunting

Children under five years of age are considered stunted when their height-for-age is 2 standard deviations below WHO's 2006 child growth standards.

Prevalence of anaemia and micronutrient deficiencies in children

Source: Micronutrient Initiative, 2009.

Values in italics are regression-based estimates as calculated by the Micronutrient Initiative. The value 0.0* is shown for countries that are assumed to be to be free of Vitamin A deficiency because they have a GDP per capita of at least $US15 000.

Anaemia

Young children (under the age of five) are considered anaemic when their haemoglobin levels are less than 110 grams per litre.

Vitamin A deficiency

Children under the age of five exhibit vitamin A deficiency when their serum retinol is less than 0.70 µmol/litre or 20 µg/dl.

Iodine deficiency
Children are considered iodine-deficient when their urinary iodine is below 100 µg/litre. Children are defined here as those aged 6–12 years.

Prevalence of obesity among adults

Sources: WHO, 2013c and United Nations, 2011b.
Regional aggregates are FAO estimates using the obesity prevalence rates presented and age-specific population weights.

Obesity
Adults over 20 years of age are considered obese when their body mass index (BMI) is greater than or equal to 30. BMI equals body weight in kilograms divided by height in metres squared (kg/m^2).

Country group and regional aggregates

The table presents country group and regional aggregates for all indicators; these are weighted averages that are calculated for the country groupings and regions as described below. In general, weighted averages for country groups are reported only when data represent at least two-thirds of the available population in that classification.

Country and regional notes

Regional and subregional groupings, as well as the designation of developing and developed regions, follow the standard country or area codes for statistical use developed by the United Nations Statistics Division (available at: unstats.un.org/unsd/methods/m49/m49.htm). Data for China exclude data for Hong Kong Special Administrative Region of China and Macao Special Administrative Region of China. Data for Sudan refer to the former sovereign state of Sudan (both Sudan and South Sudan).

ANNEX TABLE

	Prevalence of stunting among children (%)	Prevalence of micronutrient deficiencies and anaemia among children (%)			Prevalence of obesity among adults (%)
		Anaemia	Vitamin A deficiency	Iodine deficiency	
	Most recent observation	Most recent observation			2008
WORLD	**25.7**	**47.9**	**30.7**	**30.3**	**11.7**
COUNTRIES IN DEVELOPING REGIONS	**28.0**	**52.4**	**34.0**	**29.6**	**8.7**
AFRICA	**35.6**	**64.6**	**41.9**	**38.2**	**11.3**
Sub-Saharan Africa	**39.6**	**67.8**	**45.6**	**36.0**	**7.5**
Eastern Africa	**42.1**	**65.2**	**46.3**	**38.2**	**3.9**
Burundi	57.7	56.0	27.9	60.5	3.3
Comoros	46.9	*65.4*	*21.5*	..	4.4
Djibouti	32.6	*65.8*	35.2	..	10.4
Eritrea	43.7	*69.6*	*21.4*	25.3	1.8
Ethiopia	44.2	*75.2*	46.1	68.4	1.2
Kenya	35.2	69.0	84.4	36.8	4.7
Madagascar	49.2	68.3	42.1	..	1.7
Malawi	47.8	73.2	59.2	..	4.5
Mauritius	13.6	16.8	9.2	4.4	18.2
Mozambique	43.7	74.7	68.8	68.1	5.4
Réunion	..	..	..	..	..
Rwanda	44.3	41.9	6.4	0.0	4.3
Seychelles	7.7	*23.8*	*8.0*	..	24.6
Somalia	42.1	..	*61.7*	..	5.3
Uganda	38.7	64.1	27.9	3.9	4.6
United Republic of Tanzania	42.5	71.8	24.2	37.7	5.4
Zambia	45.8	52.9	54.1	72.0	4.2
Zimbabwe	32.3	19.3	35.8	14.8	8.6
Middle Africa	**35.0**	**63.9**	**56.1**	**23.8**	**4.8**
Angola	29.2	29.7	64.3	..	7.2
Cameroon	32.5	68.3	38.8	91.7	11.1
Central African Republic	40.7	84.2	68.2	79.5	3.7
Chad	38.8	*71.1*	*50.1*	29.4	3.1
Congo	31.2	*66.4*	*24.6*	..	5.3
Democratic Republic of the Congo	43.4	70.6	61.1	10.1	1.9
Equatorial Guinea	35.0	*40.8*	*13.9*	..	11.5
Gabon	26.3	*44.5*	*16.9*	38.3	15.0
Sao Tome and Principe	31.6	*36.7*	95.6	..	11.3

ANNEX TABLE *(cont.)*

	Prevalence of stunting among children *(%)*	Prevalence of micronutrient deficiencies and anaemia among children *(%)*			Prevalence of obesity among adults *(%)*
		Anaemia	Vitamin A deficiency	Iodine deficiency	
	Most recent observation	Most recent observation			2008
Northern Africa	**21.0**	**46.6**	**20.4**	**49.3**	**23.0**
Algeria	15.9	*42.5*	*15.7*	77.7	17.5
Egypt	30.7	29.9	11.9	31.2	34.6
Libya	21.0	*33.9*	*8.0*	..	30.8
Morocco	14.9	31.5	40.4	63.0	17.3
Sudan	37.9	84.6	*27.8*	62.0	6.6
Tunisia	9.0	21.7	*14.6*	26.4	23.8
Western Sahara	..	..	..	..	..
Southern Africa	**30.8**	**27.1**	**18.7**	**28.3**	**31.3**
Botswana	31.4	38.0	*26.1*	15.3	13.5
Lesotho	39.0	48.6	*32.7*	21.5	16.9
Namibia	29.6	*40.5*	*17.5*	28.7	10.9
South Africa	23.9	24.1	*16.9*	29.0	33.5
Swaziland	30.9	*46.7*	*44.6*	34.5	23.4
Western Africa	**36.4**	**77.1**	**43.5**	**40.2**	**6.6**
Benin	44.7	81.9	70.7	8.3	6.5
Burkina Faso	35.1	91.5	*54.3*	47.5	2.4
Cape Verde	21.4	*39.7*	2.0	77.4	11.5
Côte d'Ivoire	39.0	*69.0*	*57.3*	27.6	6.7
Gambia	24.4	79.4	64.0	72.8	8.5
Ghana	28.6	76.1	75.8	71.3	8.0
Guinea	40.0	79.0	*45.8*	32.4	4.7
Guinea-Bissau	32.2	*74.9*	*54.7*	..	5.4
Liberia	39.4	86.7	52.9	3.5	5.5
Mali	27.8	82.8	*58.6*	68.3	4.8
Mauritania	23.0	*68.2*	*47.7*	69.8	14.0
Niger	54.8	*81.3*	*67.0*	0.0	2.5
Nigeria	41.0	76.1	29.5	40.4	7.1
Saint Helena	..	..	..	..	..
Senegal	28.7	*70.1*	*37.0*	75.7	8.0
Sierra Leone	37.4	*83.2*	*74.8*	..	7.0
Togo	29.5	*52.4*	*35.0*	6.2	4.6
ASIA EXCLUDING JAPAN	**26.8**	**49.6**	**33.9**	**29.8**	**6.0**
Central Asia	**22.7** (A)	**38.5**	**38.3**	**39.1**	**18.4**
Kazakhstan	17.5	36.3	27.1	53.1	24.4

ANNEX TABLE *(cont.)*

	Prevalence of stunting among children *(%)*	Prevalence of micronutrient deficiencies and anaemia among children *(%)*			Prevalence of obesity among adults *(%)*
		Anaemia	Vitamin A deficiency	Iodine deficiency	
	Most recent observation	Most recent observation			2008
Kyrgyzstan	18.1	49.8	*26.3*	88.1	17.2
Tajikistan	39.2	37.7	26.8	..	9.9
Turkmenistan	28.1	35.8	*28.0*	18.7	14.3
Uzbekistan	19.6	38.1	53.1	39.8	17.3
Eastern Asia	**8.5**	**20.1**	**9.4**	**15.0**	**5.6**
China	9.4	20.0	9.3	15.7	5.6
Democratic People's Republic of Korea	32.4	31.7	*27.5*	..	3.8
Mongolia	27.5	21.4	19.8	52.8	16.4
Republic of Korea	..	16.5	0.0*	..	7.3
South-Eastern Asia	**27.4**	**41.0**	**23.4**	**30.2**	**5.3**
Brunei Darussalam	..	*24.2*	0.0*	..	7.9
Cambodia	40.9	63.4	22.3	..	2.3
Indonesia	35.6	*44.5*	*19.6*	16.3	4.7
Lao People's Democratic Republic	47.6	48.2	44.7	26.9	3.0
Malaysia	17.2	*32.4*	3.5	57.0	14.1
Myanmar	35.1	*63.2*	*36.7*	22.3	4.1
Philippines	32.3	36.3	40.1	23.8	6.4
Singapore	4.4	*18.9*	0.0*	..	6.4
Thailand	15.7	25.2	*15.7*	34.9	8.5
Timor-Leste	57.7	31.5	*45.8*	..	2.9
Viet Nam	30.5	34.1	12.0	84.0	1.6
Southern Asia	**45.5**(A)	**66.5**	**50.0**	**36.6**	**3.2**
Afghanistan	59.3	37.9	*64.5*	71.9	2.4
Bangladesh	43.2	47.0	21.7	42.5	1.1
Bhutan	33.5	80.6	22.0	13.5	5.5
India	47.9	74.3	62.0	31.3	1.9
Iran (Islamic Republic of)	7.1	*35.0*	0.5	19.7	21.6
Maldives	20.3	81.5	9.4	43.1	16.1
Nepal	40.5	78.0	32.3	27.4	1.5
Pakistan	43.0	50.9	12.5	63.6	5.9
Sri Lanka	19.2	29.9	35.3	30.0	5.0
Western Asia	**18.0**	**42.0**	**16.6**	**30.3**	**28.6**
Armenia	20.8	23.9	0.6	6.3	23.4
Azerbaijan	26.8	31.8	*32.1*	74.4	24.7
Bahrain	13.6	*24.7*	0.0*	16.2	32.6

ANNEX TABLE *(cont.)*

	Prevalence of stunting among children *(%)*	Prevalence of micronutrient deficiencies and anaemia among children *(%)*			Prevalence of obesity among adults *(%)*
		Anaemia	Vitamin A deficiency	Iodine deficiency	
	Most recent observation	Most recent observation			2008
Cyprus	..	*18.6*	0.0*	..	23.4
Georgia	11.3	*40.6*	*30.9*	80.0	21.2
Iraq	27.5	*55.9*	*29.8*	..	29.4
Israel	..	*11.8*	0.0*	..	25.5
Jordan	8.3	28.3	15.1	24.4	34.3
Kuwait	3.8	32.4	0.0*	31.4	42.8
Lebanon	16.5	28.3	*11.0*	55.5	28.2
Occupied Palestinian Territory	..	..	..	..	
Oman	9.8	50.5	5.5	49.8	22.0
Qatar	11.6	26.2	0.0*	30.0	33.1
Saudi Arabia	9.3	*33.1*	*3.6*	23.0	35.2
Syrian Arab Republic	27.5	*41.0*	*12.1*	..	31.6
Turkey	12.3	32.6	*12.4*	60.9	29.3
United Arab Emirates	..	*27.7*	0.0*	56.6	33.7
Yemen	57.7	*68.3*	*27.0*	30.2	16.7
LATIN AMERICA AND THE CARIBBEAN	**13.4**	**38.5**	**15.7**	**8.7**	**23.4**
Caribbean	**6.7**	**41.3**	**17.8**	**59.8**	**20.3**
Anguilla	..	..	..	..	..
Antigua and Barbuda	..	49.4	7.4	..	25.8
Aruba	..	..	..	..	..
Bahamas	..	*21.9*	0.0*	..	35.0
Barbados	..	*17.1*	*6.5*	..	33.4
British Virgin Islands	..	..	..	..	..
Cayman Islands	..	..	..	..	..
Cuba	7.0	*26.7*	*3.6*	51.0	20.5
Dominica	..	34.4	4.2	..	25.0
Dominican Republic	10.1	*34.6*	*13.7*	86.0	21.9
Grenada	..	*32.0*	*14.1*	..	24.0
Guadeloupe	..	..	..	..	..
Haiti	29.7	65.3	32.0	58.9	8.4
Jamaica	5.7	48.2	29.4	..	24.6
Martinique	..	..	..	..	..
Montserrat	..	..	..	..	..
Netherlands Antilles	..	..	..	..	
Puerto Rico	..	..	..	..	
Saint Kitts and Nevis	..	*22.9*	*7.1*	..	40.9
Saint Lucia	..	*32.2*	*11.3*	..	22.3
Saint Vincent and the Grenadines	..	*32.3*	2.1	..	25.1

ANNEX TABLE *(cont.)*

	Prevalence of stunting among children (%)	Prevalence of micronutrient deficiencies and anaemia among children (%)			Prevalence of obesity among adults (%)
		Anaemia	Vitamin A deficiency	Iodine deficiency	
	Most recent observation	Most recent observation			2008
Trinidad and Tobago	5.3	*30.4*	*7.2*	..	30.0
Turks and Caicos Islands	..	..	..	..	..
United States Virgin Islands	..	..	..	..	..
Central America	**18.6**	**29.6**	**22.3**	**10.1**	**30.4**
Belize	22.2	*35.9*	*11.7*	26.7	34.9
Costa Rica	5.6	20.9	8.8	8.9	24.6
El Salvador	20.6	18.4	*14.6*	4.6	26.9
Guatemala	48.0	38.1	15.8	14.4	20.7
Honduras	29.9	29.9	13.8	31.3	19.8
Mexico	15.5	29.4	26.8	8.5	32.8
Nicaragua	23.0	17.0	3.1	0.0	24.2
Panama	19.1	36.0	9.4	8.6	25.8
South America	**11.5**	**42.5**	**12.4**	**2.9**	**21.6**
Argentina	8.2	*18.1*	14.3	..	29.4
Bolivia (Plurinational State of)	27.2	51.6	*21.8*	19.0	18.9
Brazil	7.1	54.9	*13.3*	0.0	19.5
Chile	2.0	*24.4*	*7.9*	0.2	29.1
Colombia	12.7	*27.7*	5.9	6.4	18.1
Ecuador	29.0	*37.9*	*14.7*	0.0	22.0
French Guiana	..	..	..	..	..
Guyana	19.5	47.9	4.1	26.9	16.9
Paraguay	17.5	*30.2*	*14.1*	13.4	19.2
Peru	19.5	50.4	14.9	10.4	16.5
Suriname	10.7	*25.7*	*18.0*	..	25.8
Uruguay	13.9	*19.1*	*11.9*	..	23.6
Venezuela (Bolivarian Republic of)	13.4	*33.1*	*9.4*	0.0	30.8
OCEANIA EXCLUDING AUSTRALIA AND NEW ZEALAND	**35.5**	**53.8**	**11.6**	**31.8**	**22.4**
American Samoa	..	..	..	..	..
Cook Islands	..	*24.7*	*10.4*	..	64.1
Fiji	4.3	39.1	*13.6*	75.4	31.9
French Polynesia	..	..	..	..	
Guam	..	..	..	..	..
Kiribati	34.4	*41.9*	*21.8*	..	45.8
Marshall Islands	..	*30.0*	60.7	..	46.5
Micronesia (Federated States of)	..	18.7	54.2	..	42.0
Nauru	24.0	*20.0*	*10.0*	..	71.1

ANNEX TABLE *(cont.)*

	Prevalence of stunting among children (%)	Prevalence of micronutrient deficiencies and anaemia among children (%)			Prevalence of obesity among adults (%)
		Anaemia	Vitamin A deficiency	Iodine deficiency	
	Most recent observation	Most recent observation			2008
New Caledonia	..	..	..	..	..
Niue	..	*21.6*	*15.5*	..	..
Northern Mariana Islands	..	..	..	..	..
Palau	..	*22.2*	*8.9*	..	50.7
Papua New Guinea	43.9	*59.8*	11.1	27.7	15.9
Samoa	6.4	35.5	*16.1*	..	55.5
Solomon Islands	32.8	*51.7*	*13.1*	..	32.1
Tokelau	..	..	..	..	..
Tonga	2.2	*27.6*	*17.0*	..	59.6
Tuvalu	10.0	*34.2*	*21.8*	..	..
Vanuatu	25.9	*59.0*	*16.1*	..	29.8
Wallis and Futuna Islands	..	..	..	..	..
COUNTRIES IN DEVELOPED REGIONS	**7.2**	**11.8**	**3.9**	**37.7**	**22.2**
ASIA AND OCEANIA		**10.1**		**49.6**	**7.8**
Australia	..	*8.0*	0.0*	46.3	25.1
Japan	..	*10.6*	0.0*	..	4.5
New Zealand	..	*11.3*	0.0*	65.4	27.0
EUROPE		**17.0**	**6.9**	**51.2**	**21.4**
Eastern Europe		**26.0**	**14.9**	**57.5**	**23.3**
Belarus	4.5	*27.4*	*17.4*	80.9	23.4
Bulgaria	8.8	*26.7*	*18.3*	6.9	21.4
Czech Republic	2.6	*18.4*	*5.8*	47.7	28.7
Hungary	..	*18.8*	*7.0*	65.2	24.8
Poland	..	*22.7*	*9.3*	64.0	23.2
Republic of Moldova	11.3	*40.6*	*25.6*	62.0	20.4
Romania	12.8	39.8	*16.3*	46.9	17.7
Russian Federation	..	*26.5*	*14.1*	56.2	24.9
Slovakia	..	*23.4*	*8.3*	15.0	24.6
Ukraine	3.7	22.2	*23.8*	70.1	20.1
Northern Europe		**9.3**	**0.7**	**58.9**	**22.9**
Denmark	..	*9.0*	0.0*	70.8	16.2
Estonia	..	*23.4*	*8.7*	67.0	18.9
Faroe Islands	..	..	..	..	..
Finland	..	*11.5*	0.0*	35.5	19.9
Iceland	..	*7.8*	0.0*	37.7	21.9
Ireland	..	*10.3*	0.0*	60.8	24.5

ANNEX TABLE *(cont.)*

	Prevalence of stunting among children *(%)*	Prevalence of micronutrient deficiencies and anaemia among children *(%)*			Prevalence of obesity among adults *(%)*
		Anaemia	Vitamin A deficiency	Iodine deficiency	
	Most recent observation	Most recent observation			2008
Latvia	..	*26.7*	*13.0*	76.8	22.0
Lithuania	..	*23.8*	*11.1*	62.0	24.7
Norway	..	*6.4*	0.0*	..	19.8
Sweden	..	*8.6*	0.0*	..	16.6
United Kingdom	..	8.0	0.0*	..	24.9
Southern Europe		**15.8**	**4.0**	**47.3**	**20.5**
Albania	23.1	*31.0*	*18.6*	..	21.1
Andorra	..	*12.0*	0.0*	..	24.2
Bosnia and Herzegovina	11.8	*26.8*	*13.2*	22.2	24.2
Croatia	..	*23.4*	*9.2*	28.8	21.3
Gibraltar	..	..	..	..	..
Greece	..	*12.1*	0.0*	..	17.5
Holy See	..	..	..	..	..
Italy	..	*10.9*	0.0*	55.7	17.2
Malta	..	*16.3*	*4.0*	..	26.6
Montenegro	7.9	29.5	*17.2*	..	21.8
Portugal	..	*12.7*	0.0*	..	21.6
San Marino	..	*9.1*	0.0*	..	..
Serbia	6.6	29.5	*17.2*	20.8	23.0
Slovenia	..	*14.0*	0.0*	..	27.0
Spain	..	*12.9*	0.0*	50.1	24.1
The former Yugoslav Republic of Macedonia	11.5	25.8	29.7	8.7	20.3
Western Europe		**8.2**		**43.8**	**18.5**
Austria	..	*10.5*	0.0*	49.4	18.3
Belgium	..	*8.7*	0.0*	66.9	19.1
France	..	8.3	0.0*	60.4	15.6
Germany	1.3	*7.8*	0.0*	27.0	21.3
Liechtenstein	..	..	..	..	..
Luxembourg	..	*9.4*	0.0*	30.7	23.4
Monaco	..	*5.0*	0.0*	..	..
Netherlands	..	*8.7*	0.0*	37.5	16.2
Switzerland	..	*6.3*	0.0*	24.0	14.9
NORTHERN AMERICA	..	**3.5**		**15.9**	**31.0**
Bermuda	..	..	..	..	..
Canada	..	*7.6*	0.0*	..	24.3
Greenland	..	..	..	..	..
Saint Pierre and Miquelon	..	..	..	..	..
United States of America	3.9	3.1	0.0*	15.9	31.8

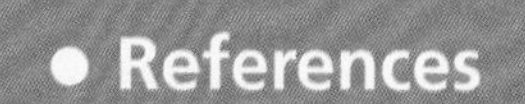

- **References**

- **Special chapters of**
  The State of Food and Agriculture

References

Acosta, A.M. 2011a. *Examining the political, institutional and governance aspects of delivering a national multi-sectoral response to reduce maternal and child malnutrition.* Analysing Nutrition Governance: Brazil Country Report. Brighton, UK, Institute of Development Studies.

Acosta, A.M. 2011b. *Analysing success in the fight against malnutrition in Peru*. IDS Working Paper No. 367. Brighton, UK, Institute of Development Studies.

Acosta, A.M. & Fanzo, J. 2012. *Fighting maternal and child malnutrition: analysing the political and institutional determinants of delivering a national multisectoral response in six countries. A synthesis paper.* Brighton, UK, Institute of Development Studies.

Afridi, F. 2011. The impact of school meals on school participation: evidence from rural India. *Journal of Development Studies*, 47: 1636–1656.

Ahmed, A., Gilligan, D., Hoddinott, J., Peterman, A. & Roy, S. 2010. *Evaluating vouchers and cash-based transfers: final inception report.* Washington, DC, IFPRI.

Akande, G.R. & Diei-Quadi, Y. 2010. *Post-harvest losses in small-scale fisheries. Case studies in five sub-Saharan African countries.* FAO Fisheries and Aquaculture Technical Paper No. 550. Rome, FAO.

Aker, J. 2008. *Does digital divide or provide? The impact of cell phones on grain markets in Niger*. Center for Global Development Working Paper No. 154. Washington, DC, Center for Global Development.

Alderman, H. & Behrman, J.R. 2004. *Estimated economic benefits of reducing low birth weight in low-income countries.* Health, Nutrition and Population Discussion Paper. Washington, DC, World Bank, Washington, DC.

Allen, L.H., Backstrand, J., Chavez, A. & Pelto, G.H. 1992. *People cannot live by tortillas alone: the results of the Mexico nutrition CRSP.* Storrs, CT, USA, University of Connecticut Department of Nutritional Sciences.

Alston, J.M., Norton, G.W. & Pardey, P.G. 1995. *Science under scarcity: principles and practice for agricultural research evaluation and priority setting*. Ithaca, NY, USA, Cornell University Press.

Alston, J.M., Sumner, D.A. & Vosti, S.A. 2006. Are agricultural policies making us fat? Likely links between agricultural policies and human nutrition and obesity, and their policy implications. *Review of Agricultural Economics*, 28(3): 313–322.

Arimond, M. & Ruel, M.T. 2002. *Progress in developing an infant and child feeding index: an example using the Ethiopia Demographic and Health Survey 2000*. Discussion Paper No. 143. Washington, DC, IFPRI.

Arimond, M. & Ruel, M.T. 2004. *Dietary diversity, dietary quality and child nutritional status: evidence from eleven demographic and health surveys*. Washington DC, Food and Nutrition Technical Assistance Project.

Arimond, M., Wiesmann, D., Becquey, E., Carriquiry, A., Daniels, M.C., Deitchler, M., Fanou-Fogny, N., Joseph, M.L., Kennedy, G., Martin-Prevel, Y. & Torheim, L.E. 2010. Simple food group diversity indicators predict micronutrient adequacy of women's diets in 5 diverse, resource-poor settings. *Journal of Nutrition*, 140(11): 2059–69.

Asfaw, A. 2007. Do government food price policies affect the prevalence of obesity? Empirical evidence from Egypt. *World Development*, 35(4): 687–701.

Attanasio, O., Battistin, E. & Mesnard, A. 2009. Food and cash transfers: evidence from Colombia. *The Economic Journal*, 122(559): 92–124.

Aworh, O.C. 2008. The role of traditional food processing technologies in national development: the West African experience. *In* G.L. Robertson & J.R. Lupien, eds. *Using food science and technology to improve nutrition and promote national development: selected case studies*, Chapter 3. Oakland, Canada, International Union of Food Science and Technology.

Ayele, Z. & Peacock, C. 2003. Improving access to and consumption of animal source foods in rural households: the experiences of a women-focused goat development program in the highlands of Ethiopia. *Journal of Nutrition*, 133: 3981S–3986S.

Barber, S. & Gertler, P. 2010. Empowering women: how Mexico's conditional cash transfer program raised prenatal care quality and birth weight. *Journal of Development Effectiveness*, 2(1): 51–73.

Barrett, C.B. & Lentz, E.C. 2010. Food insecurity. *In* R.A. Denemark, ed. *The International Studies Encyclopedia*, Vol. IV. Chichester, UK, Wiley-Blackwell.

Behrman, J.R., Calderon, M.C., Preston, S.H., Hoddinott, J., Martorell, R. & Stein, A.D. 2009. Nutritional supplementation in girls influences the growth of their children: prospective study in Guatemala. *The American Journal of Clinical Nutrition*, 90(5): 1372–1379.

Benson, T. 2008. *Improving nutrition as a development priority: addressing undernutrition in national policy processes in sub-Saharan Africa*. Research Report No. 156. Washington, DC, IFPRI.

Bezanson, K. & Isenman, P. 2010. Scaling Up Nutrition: A framework for action. *Food and Nutrition Bulletin*, 31(1): 178–186.

Berti, P., Krasevec, J. & Fitzgerald, S. 2004. A review of the effectiveness of agricultural interventions in improving nutrition outcomes. *Public Health and Nutrition*, 7(5): 599–609.

Bhutta, Z.A., Ahmed, T., Black, R.E., Cousens, S., Dewey, K., Giugliani, E., Haider, B.A., Kirkwood, B., Morris, S.S., Sachdev, H.P.S. & Shekar, M. 2008. What works? Interventions for maternal and child undernutrition and survival. *The Lancet*, 371(9610): 417–440.

Bignebat, C., Koc, A. & Lemelilleur, S. 2009. Small producers, supermarkets, and the role of intermediaries in Turkey's fresh fruit and vegetable market. *Agricultural Economics*, 40(s1): 807–816.

Birner, R., Kone, S.A., Linacre, N. & Resnick, D. 2007. Biofortified foods and crops in West Africa: Mali and Burkina Faso. *AgBioForum*, 10(3): 192–200.

Black, R.E., Allen, L.H., Bhutta, Z.A., Caulfield, L.E., de Onis, M., Ezzati, M., Mathers, C. & Rivera, J. 2008. Maternal and child undernutrition: global and regional exposures and health consequences. *The Lancet*, 371(9608): 243–260.

Block, S. 2003. *Nutrition knowledge, household coping, and the demand for micronutrient-rich foods.* Working Papers in Food Policy and Nutrition No. 20. Boston, MA, USA, Friedman School of Nutrition Science and Policy.

Block, S.A., Keiss, L., Webb, P., Kosen, S., Moench-Pfanner, R., Bloem, M.W. & Timmer, C.P. 2004, Macro shocks and micro outcomes: child nutrition during Indonesia's crisis. *Economics and Human Biology,* 2(1): 21–44.

Bloom, D.E., Cafiero, E.T., Jané-Llopis, E., Abrahams-Gessel, S., Bloom, L.R., Fathima, S., Feigl, A.B., Gaziano, T., Mowafi, M., Pandya, A., Prettner, K., Rosenberg, L., Seligman, B., Stein, A.Z. & Weinstein, C. 2011. *The global economic burden of non-communicable diseases.* Geneva, Switzerland, World Economic Forum.

Bouis, H. & Islam, Y. 2012a. *Delivering nutrients widely through biofortification: building on orange sweet potato*. Scaling up in Agriculture, rural development and nutrition, Focus 19, Brief 11. Washington, DC, IFPRI.

Bouis, H. & Islam, Y. 2012b. Biofortification: Leveraging agriculture to reduce hidden hunger. *In* S. Fan & R. Pandya-Lorch, eds. *Reshaping agriculture for nutrition and health*. Washington, DC, IFPRI.

Bouis, H.W., Eozenou, P. & Rahman, A. 2011. Food prices, household income, and resource allocation: socioeconomic perspectives on their effects on dietary quality and nutritional status. *Food and Nutrition Bulletin*, 21(1): S14–S23.

Bouis, H.E., Hotz, C., McClafferty, B., Meenakshi, J.V. & Pfeiffer, W.H. 2011. Biofortification: a new tool to reduce micronutrient malnutrition. *Food and Nutrition Bulletin*, 32(1 Suppl.): S31–40.

Bray, G.A. & Popkin, B.M. 1998. Dietary fat intake does affect obesity! *The American Journal of Clinical Nutrition*, 68(6): 1157–1173.

Broussard, N.H. 2012. Food aid and adult nutrition in rural Ethiopia. *Agricultural Economics*, 43(1): 45–59.

Brownell, K.D., Farley, T., Willett, W.C., Popkin, B.M., Chaloupka, F.J., Thompson, J.W & Ludwig, D.S. 2009. The public health and economic benefits of taxing sugar-sweetened beverages. *New England Journal of Medicine*, 361: 1599–1605.

Bryce, J., Coitinho, D., Darnton-Hill, I., Pelletier, D. & Pinstrup-Andersen, P. 2008. Maternal and child undernutrition: effective action at national level. *The Lancet*, 371(9611): 510–526.

Burch, D. & Lawrence, G., eds. 2007. *Supermarkets and agri-food supply chains: transformations in the production and consumption of foods.* Cheltenham, UK, Edward Elgar.

Burlingame, B. & Dernini, S. 2010. *Sustainable diets and biodiversity: directions and solutions for policy, research and action.* Proceedings of the International Scientific Symposium "Biodiversity and Sustainable Diets United against Hunger", 3–5 November 2010, FAO Headquarters, Rome. Rome, FAO and Bioversity International.

Caballero, B. 2007. The global epidemic of obesity: an overview. *Epidemiologic Reviews,* 29(1): 1–5.

Cadilhon, J., Moustier, P. & Poole, N. 2006. Traditional vs. modern food systems? Insights from vegetable supply chains to Ho Chi Minh City (Vietnam). *Development Policy Review*, 24(10): 31–49.

California Pan-Ethnic Health Network & Consumers Union. 2005. *Out of balance: marketing of soda, candy, snacks and fast foods drowns out healthful messages*. San Francisco, CA, USA, Consumers Union.

Cao, X.Y., Jiang, X.M., Kareem, A., Dou, Z.H., Rakeman, M.R., Zhang, M.L., Ma, T., O'Donnell, K., DeLong, N. & DeLong, G.R. 1994. Iodination of irrigation water as a method of supplying iodine to a severely iodine-deficient population in Xinjiang, China. *The Lancet*, 344(8915): 107–110.

Capacci, S. & Mazzocchi, M. 2011. Five-a-day, a price to pay: an evaluation of the UK program impact, accounting for market forces. *Journal of Health Economics*, 30(1): 87–98.

Capacci, S., Mazzocchi, M., Shankar, B., Macias, J.B., Verbeke, W., Pérez-Cueto, F.J.A., Koziol-Kozakowska, A., Piórecka, B., Niedzwiedzka, B., D'Addesa, D., Saba, A., Turrini, A., Aschemann-Witzel, J., Bech-Larsen, T., Strand, M., Smillie, L., Wills, J. & Traill, W.B. 2012. Policies to promote healthy eating in Europe: a structured review of policies and their effectiveness. *Nutrition Reviews*, 70(3): 188–200.

CDC (Centers for Disease Control and Prevention). 2012. *CDC study finds levels of trans-fatty acids in blood of U.S. white adults has decreased*. CDC Press Release, 8 February (available at http://www.cdc.gov/media/releases/2012/p0208_trans-fatty_acids.html).

Chadha, M.L., Engle, L.M., Hughes, J.d'A., Ledesma, D.R. & Weinberger, K.M. 2011. AVRDC – The World Vegetable Center's approach to alleviate malnutrition. *In* B. Thompson & L. Amoroso, eds. *Combating micronutrient deficiencies: food-based approaches*, pp. 183–197. Wallingford, UK, CAB International, and Rome, FAO.

Chou, S.Y., Rashad, I. & Grossman, M. 2008. Fast-food restaurant advertising on television and its influence on childhood obesity. *Journal of Law and Economics*, 51(4): 599–618.

Chowdhury, S., Meenakshi, J.V., Tomlins, K.I. & Owori, C. 2011. Are consumers in developing countries willing to pay more for micronutrient-dense biofortified foods? Evidence from a field experiment in Uganda. *American Journal of Agricultural Economics*, 93(1): 83–97.

Christiaensen, L., Demery, L. & Kuhl, J. 2011. The (evolving) role of agriculture in poverty reduction: an empirical perspective. *Journal of Development Economics*, 96(2): 239–254.

Coady, D.P. & Parker, S.W. 2004. Cost-effectiveness analysis of demand- and supply-side education interventions: the case of PROGRESA in Mexico. *Review of Development Economics*, 8(3): 440–451.

Colón-Ramos, U., Lindsay, A., Monge-Rojas, R., Greaney, M. & Campos, H. 2007. Translating research into action: a case study on trans fatty acid research and nutrition policy in Costa Rica. *Health Policy and Planning*, 22(6): 363–74.

Copenhagen Consensus. 2008. Copenhagen Consensus 2008 – Results. Copenhagen Consensus Center. (available at: http://www.copenhagenconsensus.com/sites/default/files/CC08_results_FINAL_0.pdf).

Cornia, G.A., Deotti, L. & Sassi, M. 2012. *Food price volatility over the last decade in Niger and Malawi: extent, sources and impact on child malnutrition*. Working Paper No. 2012-002. UNDP Regional Bureau for Africa (available at http://web.undp.org/africa/knowledge/WP-2012-002-cornia-deotti-sassi-niger-malawi.pdf).

Coulter, J. & Shepherd., A. 1995. *Inventory credit: an approach to developing agricultural market*. FAO Agricultural Services Bulletin No. 120. Rome, FAO.

Croker, H., Lucas, R. & Wardle, J. 2012. Cluster-randomised trial to evaluate the "Change for Life" mass media/ social marketing campaign in the UK. *BMC Public Health*, 12: 404.

Croppenstedt, A., Barrett, C., Carisma, B., Lowder, S., Meerman, J., Raney, T. & Thompson, B. 2013 (forthcoming). *A typology describing the multiple burdens of malnutrition*. ESA Working Paper No. 13-02. Rome, FAO.

Dar, W.D. 2004. *Macro-benefits from micronutrients for grey to green revolution in agriculture*. Paper presented at IFA International Symposium on Micronutrients, 23–25 February 2004, New Delhi, India.

Darnton-Hill, I. & Nalubola, R. 2002. Fortification strategies to meet micronutrient needs: successes and failures. *Proceedings of the Nutrition Society*, 61: 231–241.

David, C. & Otsuka, K., eds. 1994. *Modern rice technology and income distribution in Asia*. Boulder, CO, USA, Lynne Rienner Publishers.

De Boo, H. & Harding, J.E. 2006. The developmental origins of adult disease (Barker) hypothesis. *Australian and New Zealand Journal of Obstetrics and Gynaecology*, 46(1): 4–14.

de Silva, H. & Ratnadiwakara, D. 2005. The internationalization of retailing: implications for supply network restructuring in East Asia and Eastern Europe. *Journal of Economic Geography*, 5(4): 449–473.

De-Regil, L.M., Suchdev, P.S., Vist, G.E., Walleser, S. & Peña-Rosas, J.P. 2011. Home fortification of foods with multiple micronutrient powders for health and nutrition in children under two years of age. *Cochrane Database of Systematic Reviews*, 9: CD008959. Doi: 10.1002/14651858.

Deaton, A. & Drèze, J. 2009. Food and nutrition in India: facts and interpretations. *Economic & Political Weekly*, 14 February, XLIV(7): 42–65.

del Ninno, C. & Dorosh, P. 2003. Impacts of in-kind transfers on household food consumption: evidence from targeted food programmes in Bangladesh. *The Journal of Development Studies*, 40(1): 48–78.

Devaney, B. 2007. *WIC Turns 35: program effectiveness and future directions*. Paper presented at the National Invitational Conference of the Early Childhood Research Collaborative, Minneapolis, MN, USA (available at http://www.earlychildhoodrc.org/events/presentations/devaney.pdf).

Dewey, K.G. & Adu-Afarwuah, S. 2008. Systematic review of the efficacy and effectiveness of complementary feeding interventions in developing countries. *Maternal & Child Nutrition*, 4(Suppl. 1): 24–85.

Dhar, T. & Bayli, K. 2011. Fast-Food consumption and the ban on advertising targeting children: the Quebec experience. *Journal of Marketing Research*, 48(5): 799–813.

Dirven, M. & Faiguenbaum, S. 2008. The role of Santiago wholesale markets in supporting small farmers and poor consumers. *In* E. McCullough, P. Pingali & K. Stamoulis, eds. *The transformation of agrofood systems; globalization, supply chains and smallholder farmers*. Rome, FAO and London, Earthscan.

Dolan, C. & Humphrey, J. 2000. Governance and trade in fresh vegetables: the impact of UK supermarkets on the African horticulture industry. *Journal of Development Studies*, 37(2): 147–176.

Drichoutis, A., Panagiotis, L. & Nayga, R. 2006. Consumers' use of nutritional labels: a review of research studies and issues. *Academy of Marketing Science Review*, 6: 1–22.

Duflo, E. 2012. Women empowerment and economic development. *Journal of Economic Literature*, 50(4): 1051–1079.

Ecker, O., Breisinger, C. & Pauw, K. 2011. *Growth is good, but is not enough to improve nutrition*. Conference Paper No. 7. 2020 Conference: Leveraging Agriculture for Improving Nutrition and Health. 10–12 February 2011. New Delhi, India.

ESCAP (United Nations Economic and Social Commission for Asia and the Pacific). 2009. *Sustainable agriculture and food security in Asia and the Pacific*. Bangkok.

Euromonitor. 2011a. *Packaged food 2011 (Part 1). Global market performance and prospects* (available at http://www.euromonitor.com/packaged-food).

Euromonitor. 2011b. *Packaged foods in Turkey* (available at http://www.euromonitor.com/packaged-food).

Euromonitor. 2012. *Packaged foods in Mexico* (available at http://www.euromonitor.com/packaged-food).

European Commission. 2012a. *European school fruit scheme: a success story for children*. Brussels.

European Commission. 2012b. *Report from the Commission to the European Parliament and the Council in accordance with Article 184(5) of Council Regulation (EC) No. 1234/2007 on the implementation of the European School Fruit Scheme*. Brussels.

Evenson, E.R. & Rosegrant, M. 2003. The economic consequences of crop genetic improvement programmes. *In* E.R. Evenson & D. Gollin, eds. *Crop variety improvement and its effect on productivity: the impact of international agricultural research*, pp. 473–497. Wallingford, UK and Cambridge, MA, USA, CABI Publishing.

Eyles, H., Mhurchu, C.N., Nghiem, N. & Blakely, T. 2012. Food pricing strategies, population diets, and non-communicable disease: a systematic review of simulation studies. *PLoS Medicine*, 9(12): e1001353. Doi: 10.1371/journal.pmed.1001353.

Fan, S. & Pandya-Lorch, R., eds. 2012. *Reshaping agriculture for nutrition and health*. Washington, DC, IFPRI.

FAO. 2000. *Analysis of data collected in Luapula Province, Zambia by the Tropical Diseases Research Centre (TDRC) and the Food Health and Nutrition Information System (FHANIS)*. Project GCP/ZAM/052/BEL Improving Household Food and Nutrition Security in the Luapula Valley, Zambia. Rome, FAO.

FAO. 2010. *Concept note*. International Symposium on Food and Nutrition Security:

Food-Based Approaches for Improving Diets and Raising Levels of Nutrition, FAO, Rome, 7–9 December 2010. Rome.

FAO. 2011a. *Save and grow: a policymaker's guide to the sustainable intensification of smallholder crop production*. Rome.

FAO. 2011b. *The State of Food and Agriculture 2010–11: Women in agriculture: closing the gender gap for development*. Rome.

FAO. 2011c. *Evaluation of FAO's Role and Work in Nutrition. Final Report.* PC 108/6. Rome.

FAO. 2012a. *Sustainability Assessment of Food and Agriculture Systems (SAFA) 2012*. Rome.

FAO. 2012b. *Towards the future we want: end hunger and make the transition to sustainable agricultural and food systems*. Rome.

FAO. 2012c. *The State of Food and Agriculture 2012: Investing in agriculture for a better future*. Rome.

FAO. 2013. FAOSTAT statistical database (available at faostat.fao.org).

FAO & WHO. 1991. *General principles for the addition of essential nutrients to foods.* CAC/GL 9-1987 (available at http://www.codexalimentarius.org/download/standards/299/CXG_009e.pdf).

FAO & WHO. 2006. *Technical consultations on Food-Based Dietary Guidelines*. Cairo, Egypt, 6–9 December. Rome, Cairo and Alexandria, Egypt, WHO.

FAO & WHO. 2012. *Guidelines on nutrition labelling*. CAC/GL 2-1985 (available at http://www.codexalimentarius.org/download/standards/34/CXG_002e.pdf).

FAO & WFP. 2010. *The State of Food Insecurity in the World 2010: Addressing food insecurity in protracted crises*. Rome.

FAO, IFAD & WFP. 2012. *The State of Food Insecurity in the World 2012: Economic growth is necessary but not sufficient to accelerate reduction of hunger and malnutrition*. Rome.

Finkelstein, E.A., Trogdon, J.G., Cohen, J.W. & Dietz, W. 2009. Annual medical spending attributable to obesity: payer- and service-specific estimates. *Health Affairs*, 28(5): 822–831.

Finkelstein, E., Zhen, C., Nonnemaker, J. & Todd, J. 2010. Impact of targeted beverage taxes on higher- and lower-income households. *Archives of Internal Medicine*, 70(22): 2028–34.

Finucane, M.M., Stevens, G.A., Cowan, M., Danaei, G., Lin, J.K., Paciorek, C.J., Singh, G.M., Gutierrez, H., Lu, Y., Bahalim, A.N., Farzadfar, F., Riley, L.M. & Ezzati, M. 2011. National, regional and global trends in body-mass index since 1980: systematic analysis of health examination surveys and epidemiological studies with 960 country years and 9.1 million participants. *The Lancet*, 377(9765): 557–67.

Floros, J.D., Newsome, R., Fisher, W., Barbosa-Canovas, G.V., Chen, H., Dunne, C.P., German, J.B., Hall, R.L., Heldman, D.R., Karwe, M.V., Knabel, S.J., Labuza, T.P., Lund, D.B., Newell-McGloughlin, M., Robinson, J.L., Sebranek, J.G., Shewfelt, R.L., Tracy, W.F., Weaver, C.M. & Ziegler, G.R. 2010. Feeding the world today and tomorrow: the importance of food science and technology. An IFT scientific review. *Comprehensive Reviews in Food Science and Food Safety*, 9(5): 572–599.

Garde, A. 2008. Food advertising and obesity prevention: what role for the European Union? *Journal of Consumer Policy*, 31(1): 24–44.

Garrett, J. & Ersado, L. 2003. *A rural-urban comparison of cash and consumption expenditure*. Washington, DC, IFPRI. (mimeo)

Garrett, J. & Natalicchio, M., eds. 2011. *Working multisectorally in nutrition: principles, practices, and case studies.* Washington, DC, IFPRI.

Garrett, J. & Ruel, M.T. 1999. Food and nutrition in an urbanizing world. *Choices*, Special Millennium issue, fourth quarter: 12–17.

Gibson, R.S. 2011. Strategies for preventing multi-micronutrient deficiencies: a review of experiences with food-based approaches in developing countries. *In* B. Thompson & L. Amoroso, eds. 2011. *Combating micronutrient deficiencies: food-based approaches*, pp. 7–27. CAB International, Wallingford, UK and FAO, Rome, Italy.

Gibson, R. & Hotz, C. 2001. Dietary diversification/modification strategies to enhance micronutrient content and bioavailability of diets in developing countries. *British Journal of Nutrition*, 85(Suppl. 2): S159– S166.

Gibson, R., Perlas, L. & Hotz, C. 2006. Improving the bioavailability of nutrients in plant foods at the household level. *Proceedings of the Nutrition Society*, 65: 160–168.

Gill, K., Brooks, K., McDougall, J., Patel, P. & Kes, A. 2010. *Bridging the gender divide: how technology can advance women economically.* Washington, DC, International Center for Research on Women.

Gilligan, D.O., Kuman, N., McNiven, S., Meenakshi, J.V. & Quisumbing, A. 2012. *Bargaining-power and biofortification: the role of gender in adoption of orange sweet* *potato in Uganda*. Selected paper prepared for presentation at the Agricultural & Applied Economics Association's 2012 AAEA Annual Meeting, Seattle, WA, USA, 12–14 August 2012 (available at http://ageconsearch.umn.edu/bitstream/125017/2/Gilligan.pdf).

Girard, A.W., Self, J.L., McAuliffe, C. & Oludea, O. 2012. The effects of household food production strategies on the health and nutrition outcomes of women and young children: a systematic review. *Paediatric and Perinatal Epidemiology*, 26(Suppl. 1): 205–222.

Golan, E. & Unnevehr, L. 2008. Food product composition, consumer health, and public policy: introduction and overview of special section. *Food Policy*, 33(6): 465–469.

Goldman, A., Ramaswami, S. & Krider, R. 2002. Barriers to the advancement of modern food retail formats: theory and measurement. *Journal of Retailing*, 78: 281–295.

Gómez, M.I. & Ricketts, K. 2012. *Food value chains and policies influencing nutritional outcomes*. Background paper for *The State of Food and Agriculture 2013: Food systems for better nutrition*. Rome, FAO.

Gómez, M.I., Barrett, C.B., Buck, L.E., De Groote, H., Ferris, S., Gao, H.O., McCullough, E., Miller, D.D., Outhred, H., Pell, A.N., Reardon, T., Retnanestri, M., Ruben, R., Struebi, P., Swinnen, J., Touesnard, M.A., Weinberger, K., Keatinge, J.D.H., Milstein, M.B. &Yang, R.Y. 2011. Research principles for developing country food value chains. *Science*, 332(6034): 1154–1155.

Gorton, M., Sauer, J. & Supatpongkul, P.M. 2011. Wet markets, supermarkets and the "big middle" for food retailing in developing countries: evidence from Thailand. *World Development*, 39(9): 1624–1637.

Government Office for Science (United Kingdom). 2012. *Foresight report. Tackling obesities: future choices – Project report*, 2nd edition (available at: http://www.bis.gov.uk/assets/foresight/docs/obesity/17.pdf).

Greenway, F. 2006. Virus-induced obesity. *American Journal of Physiology – Regulatory, Integrative and Comparative Physiology*, 290(1): R188–R189.

Griffin, M., Sobal, J. & Lyson, T.A. 2009. An analysis of a community food waste stream. *Agriculture and Human Values*, 26(1): 67–81.

Guha-Khasnobis & James, K.S. 2010. *Urbanization and the South Asian enigma: a case study of India*. Working Paper No. 2010/37. Helsinki, United Nations University, World Institute for Development Economics Research.

Gulati, A., Minot, N., Delgado, C. & Bora, S. 2007. Growth in high-value agriculture in Asia and the emergence of vertical links with farmers. *In* J. Swinnen, ed. *Global supply chains: standards and the poor: how the globalization of food systems and standards affects rural development and poverty*, pp. 98–108. Wallingford, UK, CABI International.

Guo, X., Popkin, B.M., Mroz, T.A. & Zhai, F. 1999. Food price policy can favorably alter macronutrient intake in China. *Journal of Nutrition*, 129(5): 994–1001.

Gustavsson, J., Cederberg, C., Sonesson, U., van Otterdijk, R. & Meybeck, A. 2011. *Global food losses and food waste: extent, causes and prevention*. Rome, FAO.

Haddad, L., Alderman, H., Appleton, S., Song, L. & Yohannes, Y. 2003. Reducing child malnutrition: how far does income growth take us? *World Bank Economic Review*, 17(1): 107–131.

Harris, J. & Graff, S. 2012. Protecting young people from junk food advertising: implications for psychological research for First Amendment law. *American Journal of Public Health*, 102(2): 214–222.

HarvestPlus. 2011. *Breaking ground*. HarvestPlus Annual Report 2011. Washington, DC, HarvestPlus.

Hawkes, C. 2004. *Marketing food to children: the global regulatory environment*. Geneva, Switzerland, WHO.

Hawkes, C. 2013. *Promoting healthy diets through nutrition education and changes in the food environment: an international review of actions and their effectiveness*. Rome, FAO.

Hawkes, C., Friel, S., Lobstein, T. & Lang, T. 2012. Linking agricultural policies with obesity and noncommunicable diseases: a new perspective for a globalising world. *Food Policy*, 37(3): 343–353.

Hawkes, C., Blouin, C., Henson, S., Drager, N. & Dubes, L., eds. 2010. *Trade, food, diet and health: perspectives and policy options*. Hoboken, NJ, USA, Wiley-Blackwell.

Hayami, Y., Kikuchi, M., Moya, P.F., Bambo, L.M. & Marciano, E.B. 1978. *Anatomy of a peasant economy: a rice village in the Philippines*. Los Baños, Philippines, International Rice Research Institute.

Headey, D. 2011. *Turning economic growth into nutrition-sensitive growth*. Conference Paper No. 6. 2020 Conference on Leveraging

Agriculture for Improving Nutrition and Health, 10–12 February, New Delhi, India.

Headey, D., Chiu, A. & Kadiyala, S. 2011. *Agriculture's role in the Indian enigma: help or hindrance to the undernutrition crisis?* IFPRI Discussion Paper No. 01085. Washington, DC, IFPRI.

Helen Keller International. 2012. *Fortify West Africa: fortifying cooking oil and flour for survival and development.* Press release (available at http://www.hki.org/file/upload/HKIrelease_West_Africa_Oil_To_Flour_102307.pdf).

Herforth, A.W. 2010. *Promotion of traditional African vegetables in Kenya and Tanzania: a case study of an intervention representing emerging imperatives in global nutrition.* Ithaca, NY, USA, Cornell University.

Herforth, A. 2013. *Synthesis of guiding principles on agriculture programming for nutrition.* Rome, FAO.

Herforth, A., Jones, A. & Pinstrup-Andersen, P. 2012. *Prioritizing nutrition in agriculture and rural development projects: guiding principles for operational investments.* Health, Nutrition and Population Discussion Paper. Washington, DC, World Bank.

HLPE (High Level Panel of Experts on Food Security and Nutrition). 2012. *Social protection for food security. A report by the High Level Panel of Experts on Food Security and Nutrition.* HLPE Report No. 4. Rome.

Hoddinott, J. & Yohannes, Y. 2002. *Dietary diversity as a food security indicator.* Food Consumption and Nutrition Division Discussion Paper No. 136. Washington, DC, IFPRI.

Hoddinott, J., Maluccio, J.A., Behrman, J.R., Flores, R. & Martorell, R. 2008. Effect of a nutrition intervention during early childhood on economic productivity in Guatemalan adults. *The Lancet*, 371(9610): 411–416.

Hop, L. 2003. Programs to improve production and consumption of animal source foods and malnutrition in Vietnam. *Journal of Nutrition*, 133(11): 4006S–4009S.

Horton, S. & Ross, J. 2003. The economics of iron deficiency. *Food Policy*, 28(1): 51–75.

Horton, S., Alderman, H. & Rivera, J.A. 2008. *The challenge of hunger and malnutrition.* Copenhagen Consensus 2008, Challenge Paper. Copenhagen.

Horton, S., Mannar, V. & Wesley, A. 2008. *Micronutrient fortification (iron and salt iodization).* Working Paper. Copenhagen, Copenhagen Consensus Center.

Horton, S., Shekar, M., McDonald, C., Mahal, A. & Brooks, J.K. 2010. *Scaling up nutrition: what will it cost?* Washington, DC, World Bank.

Hotz, C. & Gibson, R. 2005. Participatory nutrition education and adoption of new feeding practices are associated with improved adequacy of complementary diets among rural Malawian children: a pilot study. *European Journal of Clinical Nutrition*, 59(2): 226–237.

Hotz, C. & Gibson, R. 2007. Traditional food-processing and preparation practices to enhance the bioavailability of micronutrients in plant-based diets. *Journal of Nutrition*, 137(4): 1097–1100.

Hotz, C., Loechl, C., de Brauw, A., Eozenou, P., Gilligan, D., Moursi, M., Munhaua, B., van Jaarsveld, P., Carriquiry, A. & Meenakshi, J.V. 2011. A large-scale intervention to introduce orange sweet potato in rural Mozambique increases vitamin A intakes among children and women. *British Journal of Nutrition*, 108(1): 163–176.

Hotz, C., Loechl, C., Lubowa, A., Tumwine, J.K., Ndeezi, G., Masawi, A.N., Baingana, R., Carriquiry, A., de Brauw, A., Meenakshi, J.V. & Gilligan, D.O. 2012. Introduction of β-carotene-rich orange sweet potato in rural Uganda results in increased vitamin A intakes among children and women and improved vitamin A status among children. *Journal of Nutrition*, 142(10): 1871-80.

Iannotti, L., Cunningham, K. & Ruel, M. 2009. *Improving diet quality and micronutrient nutrition: homestead food production in Bangladesh.* IFPRI Discussion Paper No. 00928. Washington, DC, IFPRI.

IDS (Institute of Development Studies). 2012. *Accelerating reductions in undernutrition: what can nutrition governance tell us?* IDS in Focus Policy Briefing, Issue 22. Brighton, UK.

IFAD (International Fund for Agricultural Development). 2003. *Agricultural marketing companies as sources of smallholder credit in Eastern and Southern Africa: experiences, insights and potential donor role.* Rome.

INCAP (Instituto de Nutrición de Centroamérica y Panamá). 2013. *Mejor compra.* Webpage (available at www.incap.int/sisvan/index.php/es/areas-tematicas/metodologias-de-apoyo/mejor-compra).

Imdad, A., Yakoob, M.Y. & Bhutta, Z.A. 2011. Impact of maternal education about complementary feeding and provision of complementary foods on child growth in developing countries. *BMC Public Health*, 11(Suppl. 3): S25.

Ippolito, P.M. & Mathias, A.D. 1993. Information, advertising, and health choices: a study of the cereal market. *Rand Journal of Economics*, 21(3): 459–480.

Ivers, L.C., Cullen, K.A., Freedberg, K.A., Block, S., Coates, J., Webb, P. & Mayer, K.H. 2009. HIV/AIDS, undernutrition, and food insecurity. *Clinical Infectious Diseases*, 49(7): 1096–1102.

Jabbar, M.A. & Admassu, S.A. 2010. Assessing consumer preferences for quality and safety attributes of food in the absence of official standards: the case of beef, raw milk and local butter in Ethiopia. *In* M.A. Jabbar, D. Baker & M.L. Fadiga, eds. *Demand for livestock products in developing countries with a focus on quality and safety attributes: evidence from Asia and Africa*, pp. 38–58. ILRI Research Report 24. Nairobi, International Livestock Research Institute.

Jabbar, M.A., Baker, D. & Fadiga, M.L., eds. 2010. *Demand for livestock products in developing countries with a focus on quality and safety attributes: evidence from Asia and Africa*. ILRI Research Report 24. Nairobi, International Livestock Research Institute.

Jame, P.C. & Lock, K. 2009. Do school based food and nutrition policies improve diet and reduce obesity? *Preventive Medicine*, 48(1): 45–53.

Jayne, T.S., Mason, N., Myers, R., Ferris, J., Mather, D., Sitko, N., Beaver, M., Lenski, N., Chapoto, A. & Boughton, D. 2010. *Patterns and trends in food staples markets in Eastern and Southern Africa: toward the identification of priority investments and strategies for developing markets and promoting smallholder productivity growth*. MSU International Development Working Paper No. 104. East Lansing, MI, USA, Michigan State University.

Kaplinsky, R. & Morris, M. 2001. *A handbook for value chain research*. Ottawa, Canada, International Development Research Centre.

Keith, S.W., Redden, D.T., Katzmarzyk, P.T., Boggiano, M.M., Hanlon, E.C., Benca, R.M., Ruden, D., Pietrobelli, A., Barger, J.L., Fontaine, K.R., Wang, C., Aronne, L.J., Wright, S.M., Baskin, M., Dhurandhar, N.V., Lijoi, M.C., Grilo, C.M., DeLuca, M., Westfall, A.O. & Allison, D.B. 2006. Putative contributors to the secular increase in obesity: exploring the roads less travelled. *International Journal of Obesity*, 30(11): 1585–1594.

Keller, S.K. & Schulz, P.J. 2011. Distorted food pyramid in kids programs: a content analysis of television advertising watched in Switzerland. *European Journal of Public Health*, 21(3): 300–305.

Kennedy, E. 2004. Dietary diversity, diet quality, and body weight regulation. *Nutrition Reviews*, 62(7): S78–S81.

Kennedy, E. & Bouis, H.E. 1993. *Linkages between agriculture and nutrition: implications for policy and research*. Washington, DC, IFPRI.

Kes, A. & Swaminathan, H. 2006. Gender and time poverty in sub-Saharan Africa. *In* C.M. Blackden & Q. Wodon, eds. *Gender, time use, and poverty in sub-Saharan Africa*, pp. 13–38. World Bank Working Paper No. 73. Washington, DC, World Bank.

Kirksey, A., Harrison, G.G., Galal, O.M., McCabe, G.A., Wachs, T.D. & Rahmanifar, A. 1992. *The human cost of moderate malnutrition in an Egyptian village. Final Report Phase II: Nutrition CRSP*. Lafayette, LA, USA, Purdue University.

Kuchler, F., Tegene, A. & Harris, J.M. 2004. Taxing snack foods: what to expect for diet and tax revenues. *Current issues in economics of food markets*. Agriculture Information Bulletin No. 747–08. Washington, DC, United States Department of Agriculture, Economic Research Service.

Kumar, S.K. 1987. The nutrition situation and its food policy links. *In* J.W. Mellor, C.L. Delgado & M.J. Blackie, eds. *Accelerating food production in sub-Saharan Africa*, pp. 39–52. Baltimore, MD, USA, The Johns Hopkins University Press for IFPRI.

Kumar, N. & Quisumbing, A.R. 2011. Access, adoption, and diffusion: understanding the long-term impacts of improved vegetable and fish technologies in Bangladesh. *Journal of Development Effectiveness*, 3(2): 193–219.

Lentz, E.C. & Barrett, C.B. 2007. Improving food aid: What reforms would yield the highest payoff? *World Development*, 36(7): 1152–1172.

Lentz, E.C. & Barrett, C.B. 2012. The economics and nutritional impacts of food assistance policies and programmes. Background paper for *The State of Food and Agriculture 2013: Food systems for better nutrition*. Rome, FAO.

Lim, S.S. *et al.*, 2012. A comparative risk assessment of burden of disease and injury attributable to 67 risk factors and risk factor clusters in 21 regions, 1990–2010: a systematic analysis for the Global Burden of Disease Study 2010. *The Lancet*, 380(9859): 2224–60.

Lippe, R., Seens, H. & Isvilanonda, S. 2010. Urban household demand for fresh fruits and vegetables in Thailand. *Applied Economics Journal*, 17(1): 1–26.

Lobstein, T. & Frelut, M-L. 2003. Prevalence of overweight among children in Europe. *Obesity Reviews*, 4(4): 195–200.

Lyimo, M.H., Nyagwegwe, S. & Mnkeni, A.P. 1991. Investigations on the effect of traditional food processing, preservation and storage methods on vegetable nutrients: a case study in Tanzania. *Plant Foods for Human Nutrition*, 41(1): 53–57.

Ma, G., Jin, Y., Li, Y., Zhai, F., Kok, F.K., Jacobsen, E. & Yang, X. 2007. Iron and zinc deficiencies in China: what is a feasible and cost-effective strategy? *Public Health Nutrition*, 11(6): 632–638.

Margolies, A. & Hoddinott, J. 2012. *Mapping the impacts of food aid: current knowledge and future directions.* Working Paper No. 2012/34. Helsinki, United Nations University, World Institute for Development Economics Research.

Martínez, R. & Fernández, A. 2008. *The cost of hunger: social and economic impact of child undernutrition in Central America and the Dominican Republic.* Santiago, Economic Commission for Latin America and the Caribbean (ECLAC) and WFP.

Mason, J.B., Chotard, S., Cercone, E., Dieterich, M., Oliphant, N.P., Mebrahtu, S. & Hailey, P. 2010. Identifying priorities for emergency intervention from child wasting and mortality estimates in vulnerable areas of the Horn of Africa. *Food and Nutrition Bulletin*, 31(3): S234–S247.

Masset, E., Haddad, L., Cornelius, A. & Isaza-Castro, J. 2011. *A systematic review of agricultural interventions that aim to improve nutritional status of children.* London, EPPI-Centre, Social Science Research Unit, Institute of Education, University of London.

Mayer, A.B., Latham, M.C., Duxbury, J.M., Hassan, N. & Frongillo, E.A. 2011. A food systems approach to increase dietary zinc intake in Bangladesh based on an analysis of diet, rice production and processing. *In* B. Thompson & L. Amoroso, eds. *Combating micronutrient deficiencies: food-based approaches*, pp. 254–267. Wallingford, UK, CAB International, and Rome, FAO.

Mazzocchi, M., Traill, W.B. & Shogren, J.F. 2009. *Fat economics.* Oxford, UK, Oxford University Press.

Mazzocchi, M., Shankar, B. & Traill, B. 2012. *The development of global diets since ICN 1992: influences of agri-food sector trends and policies.* FAO Commodity and Trade Policy Research Working Paper No. 34. Rome, FAO.

McKinsey. 2007. Selling to "mom-and-pop" stores in emerging markets. *McKinsey Quarterly*, March (Special edition) (available at http://www.mckinseyquarterly.com/Marketing/Strategy/Selling_to_mom-and-pop_stores_in_emerging_markets_1957).

McNulty, J. 2013. *Challenges and issues in nutrition education.* Background paper for the International Conference on Nutrition (ICN2). Rome, FAO.

MDG Achievement Fund. 2013. *Children, food security and nutrition. MDG-F thematic study: review of key findings and achievements.* New York, USA, United Nations.

Meenakshi, J.V., Banerji, A., Manyong, V., Tomlins, K., Mittal, N. & Hamukwala, P. 2012. Using a discrete choice experiment to elicit the demand for a nutritious food: willingness-to-pay for orange maize in rural Zambia. *Journal of Health Economics*, 31(1): 62–71.

Menon, P., Ruel, M.T. & Morris, S.S. 2000. Socio-economic differentials in child stunting are consistently larger in urban than in rural areas. *Food and Nutrition Bulletin*, 21(3): 282–9.

Mergenthaler, M., Weinberger, K. & Qaim, M. 2009. Consumer valuation of food quality and food safety attributes in Vietnam. *Review of Agricultural Economics*, 31(2): 266–283.

Meyer, J. 2007. *The use of cash/vouchers in response to vulnerability and food insecurity.* Rome, WFP.

Micronutrient Initiative. 2009. *Investing in the future: a united call to action on vitamin and mineral deficiencies. Global report 2009.* Ottawa, Canada.

Miller, D. & Welch, R. 2012. *Food system strategies for preventing micronutrient malnutrition.* Background paper for *The State of Food and Agriculture 2013: Food systems for better nutrition*. Rome, FAO.

Minten, B. 2008. The food retail revolution in poor countries: is it coming or is it over? *Development and Cultural Change*, 56(4): 767–789.

Minten, B. & Barrett, C.B. 2008. Agricultural technology, productivity, and poverty in Madagascar. *World Development*, 36(5): 797–822.

Minten, B. & Reardon, T. 2008. Food prices, quality, and quality's pricing in supermarkets versus traditional markets in developing countries. *Review of Agricultural Economics*, 30(3): 480–490.

Mohmand, S.K. 2012. *Policies without politics: analysing nutrition governance in India*. Analysing Nutrition Governance: India Country Report. Brighton, UK, Institute of Development Studies.

Monteiro, C.A. & Cannon, G. 2012. The impact of transnational "big food" companies on the South: a view from Brazil. *PloS Medicine*, 9(7): e1001252.

Moretti, D., Zimmermann, M.B., Muthayya, S., Thankachan, P., Lee, T.C., Kurpad, A.V. & Hurrell, R.F. 2006. Extruded rice fortified with micronized ground ferric pyrophosphate reduces iron deficiency in Indian schoolchildren: a double-blind randomized controlled trial. *The American Journal of Clinical Nutrition*, 84(4): 822–829.

Mozaffarian, D., Afshin, A., Benowitz, N.L., Bittner, V., Daniels, S.R., Franch, H.A., Jacobs, D.R., Kraus, W.E., Kris-Etherton, P.M., Krummel, D.A., Popkin, B.M., Whitsel, L.P. & Zakai, N.A. 2012. Population approaches to improve diet, physical activity, and smoking habits: a scientific statement from the American Heart Association. *Circulation*, 126(12): 1514–1563.

Murphy, S.P., Gewa, C., Liang, L.J., Grillenberger, M., Bwibo, N.O. & Neumann, C.G. 2003. School snacks containing animal source foods improve dietary quality for children in rural Kenya. *The Journal of Nutrition*, 133: 3950S–3956S.

Namugumya, B.S. 2012. Advocacy to reduce malnutrition in Uganda: some lessons for sub-Saharan Africa. *In* S. Fan & R. Pandya-Lorch, eds. *Reshaping agriculture for nutrition and health*, pp. 163–171. Washington, DC, IFPRI.

National Institute for Health and Clinical Excellence. 2007. *Obesity: the prevention, identification, assessment and management of overweight and obesity in adults and children*, Appendix 5 (available at http://www.nice.org.uk/guidance/index.jsp?action=download&o=38284).

National Obesity Observatory. 2009. *Body Mass Index as a measure of obesity* (available at http://www.noo.org.uk/securefiles/130511_1911//noo_BMI.pdf).

Neumann, C.G., Bwibo, N.O. & Sigman, M. 1992. *Final Report Phase II: Functional implications of malnutrition, Kenya Project. Nutrition CRSP.* Los Angeles, CA, USA, University of California, Los Angeles.

Neumann, C.G., Bwibo, N.O., Murphy, S.P., Sigman, M., Whaley, S., Allen, L.H., Guthrie, D., Weiss, R.E. & Demment, M.W. 2003. Animal source foods improve dietary quality, micronutrient status, growth and cognitive function in Kenyan school children: background, study design and baseline findings. *The Journal of Nutrition*, 133(11 Suppl. 2): 3941S–3949S.

Neven, D., Reardon, T., Chege, J. & Wang, H. 2005. *Supermarkets and consumers in Africa: the case of Nairobi, Kenya.* Staff Paper No. 2005-04. East Lansing, MI, USA, Department of Agricultural Economics, Michigan State University.

Nishida, C. 2004. Appropriate body-mass index for Asian populations and its implications for policy and intervention strategies: WHO Expert Consultation. *The Lancet*, 363(9403): 157–163.

Nnoaham, K.E., Sacks, G., Rayner, M., Mytton, O. & Gray, A. 2009. Modelling income group differences in the health and economic impacts of targeted food taxes and subsidies. *International Journal of Epidemiology*, 38(5): 1324–1333.

Nubé, M. & Voortman, R.L. 2011. Human micronutrient deficiencies: linkages with micronutrient deficiencies in soils, crops and animal nutrition. *In* B. Thompson & L. Amoroso, eds. *Combating micronutrient deficiencies: food-based approaches*, pp. 289–311. Wallingford, UK, CAB International, and Rome, FAO.

Nugent, R. 2011. *Bringing agriculture to the table: how agriculture and food can play a role in preventing chronic disease*. Chicago, IL, USA, The Chicago Council on Global Affairs.

Pinstrup-Andersen, P. & Watson II, D.D. 2011. *Food policy for developing countries: the role of government in global, national, and local food systems*. Ithaca, NY, USA, Cornell University Press.

Pollard, C., Miller, M., Daly, A.M., Crouchley, K., O'Donoghue, K.J., Lang, A.J. & Binns, C.W. 2008. Increasing fruit and vegetable consumption: success of the Western Australian Go for 2&5 campaign. *Public Health Nutrition*, 11(3): 314–320.

Popkin, B.M., Adair, L.S. & Ng, S.W. 2012. Global nutrition transition and the pandemic of obesity in developing countries. *Nutrition Reviews*, 70(1): 3–21.

Popkin, B.M., Kim, S., Rusev, E.R., Du, S. & Zizza, C. 2006. Measuring the full economic costs of diet, physical activity and obesity-related chronic diseases. *Obesity Reviews*, 7(3): 271–293.

Powell, L.M., Auld, M.C., Chaloupka, F.J., O'Malley, P.M. & Johnston, L.D. 2007. Access to fast food and food prices: relationship with fruit and vegetable consumption and overweight among adolescents. *In* K. Bolin & J. Cawley, eds. *Advances in Health Economics and Health Services Research. Vol. 17, The economics of obesity,* pp. 23–48. Bingley, UK, Emerald Publishing.

Qaim, M., Stein, A.J. & Meenakshi, J.V. 2007. Economics of biofortification, *Agricultural Economics*, 37(s1): 119–133.

Quisumbing, A.R., ed. 2003. *Household decisions, gender, and development: a synthesis of recent research*. Washington, DC, IFPRI.

Quisumbing, A. & Pandolfelli, L. 2010. Promising approaches to address the needs of the poor female farmers: Resources, constraints, and interventions. *World Development*, 38(4): 581–592.

Rahkovsky, I., Martinez, S. & Kuchler, F. 2012. *New food choices free of trans fats better align U.S. diets with health recommendations*. Economic Information Bulletin No. 95. Washington, DC, United States Department of Agriculture, Economic Research Service.

Reardon, T. & Barrett, C. 2000. Agroindustrialization, globalization, and international development: an overview of issues, patterns, and determinants. *Agricultural Economics*, 23(3): 195–205.

Reardon, T. & Gulati, A. 2008. *The rise of supermarkets and their development implications: international experience relevant for India*. IFPRI Discussion Paper No. 00752. Washington, DC, IFPRI.

Reardon, T. & Minten, B. 2011. *The quiet revolution in India's food supply chains.* IFPRI Discussion Paper No. 01115. Washington, DC, IFPRI.

Reardon, T. & Timmer, P. 2007. Transformation of agricultural output in developing countries since 1950: how has thinking changed? *In* R.E. Evenson, P. Pingali & T.P Schultz, eds. *Handbook of agricultural economics. Vol. 3, Agricultural development: farmers, farm production and farm markets*, Chapter 13. Amsterdam, North-Holland.

Reardon, T. & Timmer, C.P. 2012. The Economics of the Food System Revolution. *The Annual Review of Resource Economics*, 4: 225–264.

Reardon, T., Henson, S. & Gulati, A. 2010. Links between supermarkets and food prices, diet diversity and food safety in developing countries. *In* C. Hawkes, C. Blouin, S. Henson, N. Drager & L. Dube, eds. *Trade, food, diet and health: perspectives and policy options.* Hoboken, NJ, USA, Wiley-Blackwell.

Reddy, G., Murthy, M. & Meena, P. 2010. Value chains and retailing of fresh vegetables and fruits, Andhra Pradesh. *Agricultural Economics Research Review*, 23(Conference): 435–460.

Regmi, A. & Gehlhar, M., eds. 2005. *New directions in global food markets*. Agriculture Information Bulletin No. 794. Washington, DC, United States Department of Agriculture.

Regmi, A., Deepak, M.S., Seale Jr., J.L. & Bernstein, J. 2001. Cross-country analysis of food consumption patterns. *In* A. Regmi, ed. *Changing structure of global food consumption and trade*, pp. 14–22. Agriculture and Trade Reports, WRS-01-1. Washington, DC, United States Department of Agriculture, Economic Research Service.

Ren, Q., Fan, F., Zhang, Z., Zheng, X. & DeLong, G.R. 2008. An environmental approach to correcting iodine deficiency: supplementing iodine in soil by iodination of irrigation water in remote areas. *Journal of Trace Elements in Medicine and Biology*, 22(1): 1–8.

Renkow, M., Hallstrom, D. & Karanja, D. 2004. Rural infrastructure, transaction costs, and market participation in Kenya. *Journal of Development Economics*, 73(1): 349–367.

Robberstadt, B. 2005. QALYs vs DALYs vs LYs gained: what are the differences, and what difference do they make for health care priority setting? *Norsk Epidemiologi*, 15(2): 183–191.

Rodrigues, J. & Baker, G.A. 2012. Grameen Danone Foods Limited (GDF). *International Food and Agribusiness Management Review*, 15(1): 127–158.

Rosenheck, R. 2008. Fast food consumption and increased caloric intake: a systematic review of a trajectory towards weight gain and obesity risk. *Obesity Reviews*, 9(6): 535–547.

Ruben, R., van Tilburg, A., Trienekens, J. & van Boekel, M. 2007. Linking market integration, supply chain governance, quality, and value added in tropical food chains. *In* R. Ruben, M. van Boekel, A. van Tilburg & J. Trienekens, eds. *Tropical food chains: governance regimes for quality management*, pp. 13–46. Wageningen, Netherlands, Wageningen Academic Publishers.

Ruel, M.T. 2000. Urbanization in Latin America: constraints and opportunities for child feeding and care. *Food and Nutrition Bulletin*, 21(1): 12–24.

Ruel, M.T. 2003. Operationalizing dietary diversity: a review of measurement issues and research priorities. *Journal of Nutrition*, 133(11 Suppl. 2): 3911S–3926S.

Ruel, M.T., Garrett, J., Morris, S.S., Maxwell, D., Oshaug, O., Engle, P., Menon, P., Slack, A. & Haddad, L. 1998. *Urban challenges to food and nutrition security: a review of food security, health, and caregiving in the cities.* Food Consumption and Nutrition Division Discussion Paper No. 51. Washington, DC, IFPRI.

Ryckembusch, D., Frega, R., Silva, M.G., Gentilini, U., Sandogo, I., Grede, N. & Brown, L. 2013. Enhancing nutrition: a new tool for *ex-ante* comparison of commodity-based vouchers and food transfers. *World Development* (in press, corrected proof, available at http://dx.doi.org/10.1016/j.worlddev.2013.01.021).

Sadler, K., Mitchard, E., Abdi, A., Shiferaw, Y., Bekele, G. & Catley, A. 2012. *Milk matters: the impact of dry season livestock support on milk supply and child nutrition in Somali Region, Ethiopia*. Somerville, MA, USA, Feinstein International Center, Tufts University, and Addis Ababa, Save the Children.

Schäfer Elinder, L. 2005. Obesity, hunger, and agriculture: the damaging role of subsidies. *British Medical Journal*, 331(7528): 1333–1336.

Schaetzel, T. & Sankar, R. 2002. Effects of micronutrient deficiencies on human health: its status in South Asia. *Journal of Crop Production*, 6(1/2): 55–98.

Schipmann, C. & Qaim, M. 2010. Spillovers from modern supply chains to traditional markets: product innovation and adoption by smallholders. *Agricultural Economics*, 41(3/4): 361–371.

Schipmann, C. & Qaim, M. 2011. Modern food retailers and traditional markets in developing countries: comparing quality, prices, and competition strategies in Thailand. *Applied Economic Perspectives and Policy*, 33(3): 345–362.

Schmidhuber, J. 2007. *The EU diet: evolution, evaluation and impacts of the CAP*. Paper presented at the WHO Forum on "Trade and healthy food and diets", Montreal, Canada, 7–13 November 2007 (available at http://www.fao.org/fileadmin/templates/esa/Global_persepctives/Presentations/Montreal-JS.pdf).

Schoonover, H. & Muller, M. 2006. *Food without thought: how U.S. farm policy contributes to obesity*. Minneapolis, MN, USA, Institute for Agriculture and Trade Policy.

Sharma, V.P. 2012. *Food subsidy in India: trends, causes and policy reform options*. Working Paper No. 2012-08-02. Ahmedabad, India, Indian Institute of Management.

Sherman, J. & Muehlhoff, E. 2007. Developing a nutrition and health education program for primary schools in Zambia. *Journal of Nutrition Education and Behavior*, 39(6): 335–342.

Shi, L. & Zhang, J. 2011. Recent evidence of the effectiveness of educational interventions for improving complementary feeding practices in developing countries. *Journal of Tropical Pediatrics*, 57(2): 91–98.

Shimokawa, S. 2010. Nutrient intake of the poor and its implications for the nutritional effect of cereal price subsidies: evidence from China. *World Development*, 38(7): 1001–1011.

Signal, L., Lanumata, T., Robinson, J.-A., Tavila, A., Wilton, J. & Ni Mhurchu, C. 2007. Perceptions of New Zealand nutrition labels by Māori, Pacific and low-income shoppers. *Public Health Nutrition*, 11(7): 706–713.

Silva-Barbeau, I., Hull, S.G., Prehm, M.S. & Barbeau, W.E. 2005. Women's access to food-processing technology at the household level is associated with improved diets at the pre-harvest lean season in The Gambia. *Food and Nutrition Bulletin*, 26(3): 297–308.

Singh, S.P., Puna Ji Gite, L. & Agarwal, N. 2006. Improved farms tools and equipment for women workers for increased productivity and reduced drudgery. *Gender, Technology and Development*, 12(2): 229–244.

Siu, Wai-sum & Man-yi Tsoi, T. 1998. Nutrition label usage of Chinese consumers. *British Food Journal*, 100(1): 25–29.

Smith, L.C., Ruel, M.T. & Ndiaye, A. 2005. Why is child malnutrition lower in urban than in rural areas? Evidence from 36 developing countries. *World Development*, 33(8): 1285–1305.

Smith, L.C., Ramakrishnan, U., Ndiaye, A., Haddad, L. & Martorell, R. 2003. *The importance of women's status for child nutrition in developing countries.* Research Report No. 131. Washington, DC, IFPRI.

Socialinnovator. 2012. *Grameen-Danone Partnership, Bangladesh*. Webpage (available at: http://socialinnovator.info/ways-supporting-social-innovation/market-economy/social-business-partnerships/partnerships-betweeen/grameen-danone-partnership-b).

Stein, A.J. & Qaim, M. 2007. The human and economic cost of hidden hunger. *Food and Nutrition Bulletin*, 28(2): 125–134.

Stein, A.J., Meenakshi, J.V., Qaim, M., Nestel, P., Sachdev, H.P.S. & Bhutta, Z.A. 2005. *Analyzing the health benefits of biofortified staple crops by means of the disability adjusted life years approach: a handbook focusing on iron, zinc and vitamin A.* HarvestPlus Technical Monograph 4. Washington, DC, IFPRI.

Stevens, G.A., Singh, G.M., Lu, Y., Danaei, G., Lin, J.K., Finucane, M.M., Bahalim, A.N. *et al.* 2012. National, regional, and global trends in adult overweight and obesity prevalences. *Population Health Metrics*, 10: 22 (available at http://www.pophealthmetrics.com/content/10/1/22).

Strom, S. 2012. "Fat tax" in Denmark is repealed after criticism. *New York Times*, 12 November (available at http://www.nytimes.com/2012/11/13/business/global/fat-tax-in-denmark-is-repealed-after-criticism.html?_r=0).

Stuckler, D. & Nestle, M. 2012. Big food, food systems, and global health. *PLoS Medicine*, 9(6): e1001242

Suárez, S.P. 2011. Disability-adjusted Life Years (DALYs): a methodology for conducting economic studies of food-based interventions such as biofortification. *In* B. Thompson & L. Amoroso, eds. *Combating micronutrient deficiencies: food-based approaches*, pp. 366–379. Wallingford, UK, CAB International, and Rome, FAO.

Swinnen, J. & Maertens, M. 2006. *Globalization, privatization and vertical coordination in food value chains in developing and transition countries.* Paper prepared for International Association of Agricultural Economics, Queensland, Australia, 12–18 August 2006 (available at http://ageconsearch.umn.edu/bitstream/25626/1/pl06sw01.pdf).

Taylor, L. 2012a. *The nutrition agenda in Bangladesh: "Too massive to handle?" Analysing Nutrition Governance: Bangladesh Country Report.* Brighton, UK, Institute of Development Studies.

Taylor, L. 2012b. *A second chance: focusing Zambia's nutrition sector in the context of political change. Analysing Nutrition Governance: Zambia Country Report.* Brighton, UK, Institute of Development Studies.

Thompson, B. & Amoroso, L., eds. 2011. *Combating micronutrient deficiencies: food-based approaches.* Wallingford, UK, CAB International, and Rome, FAO.

Thorne-Lyman, A.L., Valpiani, N., Sun, K., Semba, R.D., Klotz, C.L., Kraemer, K., Akhter, N., de Pee, S., Moench-Pfanner, R. & Sari, M. 2010. Household dietary diversity and food expenditures are closely linked in rural Bangladesh, increasing the risk of malnutrition due to the financial crisis. *Journal of Nutrition*, 140(1): 182–188.

Tontisirin, K., Nantel, G. & Bhattacharjeef, L. 2002. Food-based strategies to meet the challenges of micronutrient malnutrition in the developing world. *Proceedings of the Nutrition Society*, 61(2): 243–250.

Tschirley, D., Ayieko, M., Hichaambwa, M., Goeb, J. & Loescher, W. 2010. *Modernizing Africa's fresh produce supply chains without rapid supermarket takeover: towards a definition of research and investment priorities.* MSU International Development Working Paper No. 106. East Lansing, MI, USA, Michigan State University, Department of Agricultural, Food, and Resource Economics and Department of Economics.

UNEP (United Nations Environment Programme). 2012. *Avoiding future famines: strengthening the ecological foundation of food security through sustainable food systems.* Nairobi.

UNICEF (United Nations Children's Fund). 2013. Statistics by area/Child nutrition/Underweight disparities. *Childinfo: Monitoring the situation of women and children* (available at: http://www.childinfo.org/malnutrition_weightbackground.php).

UNICEF & The Micronutrient Initiative. 2004. *Vitamin and mineral deficiencies: a global progress report.* Ottawa, Canada.

UNICEF, WHO & The World Bank. 2012. *Levels and trends in child malnutrition: Joint child malnutrition estimates.* New York, USA, UNICEF, Geneva, Switzerland, WHO and Washington, DC, World Bank.

United Nations. 2011a. *Political declaration of the High-level Meeting of the General Assembly on the Prevention and Control of Non-communicable Diseases.* Document A/66/L.1 (available at http://www.un.org/ga/search/view_doc.asp?symbol=A/66/L.1).

United Nations. 2011b. Annual population by five-year age groups 1950–2010 – both sexes. *World Population Prospects, the 2010 Revision* (available at http://esa.un.org/wpp/Excel-Data/population.htm).

United Nations. 2012. National Accounts Main Aggregates Database (available at http://unstats.un.org/unsd/snaama/introduction.asp).

Unnevehr, L.J. & Jagmanaite, E. 2008. Getting rid of trans fats in the U.S. Diet: Policies, incentives, and progress. *Food Policy*, 33(6): 497–503.

UNSCN (United Nations Standing Committee on Nutrition). 2010. *Sixth report on the world nutrition situation: progress in nutrition.* Geneva, Switzerland.

USDA (United States Department of Agriculture). 2009. *About EFNEP*. Webpage (available at www.nifa.usda.gov/nea/food/efnep/about.html).

USDA. 2012. *National School Lunch Program.* Fact sheet (available at http://www.fns.usda.gov/slp).

Vaitla, B., Devereux, S. & Swan, S.H. 2009. Seasonal hunger: a neglected problem with proven solutions. *PLoS Medicine*, 6(6): e1000101.

Van de Poel, E., O'Donnell, O. & Van Doorslaer, E. 2007. Are urban children really healthier? Evidence from 47 developing countries. *Social Science & Medicine*, 65(10): 1986–2003.

van Jaarsveld, P.J., Faber, M., Tanumihardjo, S.A., Nestel, P., Lombard, C.J. & Benadé, A.J.S. 2005. ß-Carotene-rich orange-fleshed sweet potato improves the vitamin A status of primary school children assessed with the modified-relative-dose-response test. *The American Journal of Clinical Nutrition*, 81(5): 1080–1087.

Variyam, J. 2007. Do nutrition labels improve dietary outcomes? *Health Economics*, 17(6): 695–708.

Veerman, J.L., Van Beeck, E.F., Barendregt, J.J. & Mackenbach, J.P. 2009. By how much would limiting TV food advertising reduce childhood obesity? *European Journal of Public Health*, 19(4): 365–369.

Victora, C.G., Adair, L., Fall, C., Hallal, P.C., Martorell, R., Richter, L. & Sachdev, H.S. for the Maternal and Child Undernutrition Study Group. 2008. Maternal and child undernutrition: consequences for adult health and human capital. *The Lancet*, 371(9609): 340–57.

Wanyoike, F., Kaitibie, S., Kuria, S., Bruntse, A., Thendiu, I.N., Mwangi, D.M. & Omore, A. 2010. Consumer preferences and willingness to pay for improved quality and safety: the case of fresh camel milk and dried camel meat (nyir nyir) in Kenya. *In* M.A. Jabbar, D. Baker & M.L. Fadiga, eds. *Demand for livestock products in developing countries with a focus on quality and safety attributes: evidence from Asia and Africa*, pp. 93–102. ILRI Research Report 24. Nairobi, International Livestock Research Institute.

Waters, B.M. & Sankaran, R.P. 2011. Moving micronutrients from the soil to the seeds: genes and physiological processes from a biofortification perspective. *Plant Science*, 180: 562–574.

Webb, P. & Block, S. 2004. Nutrition information and formal schooling as inputs to child nutrition. *Economic Development and Cultural Change*, 52(4): 801–820.

Webb, P., Rogers, B., Rosenberg, I., Schlossman, N., Wanke, C., Bagriansky, J., Sadler, K., Johnson, Q., Tilahun, J., Reese Masterson, A. & Narayan, A. 2011. *Delivering improved nutrition: recommendations for changes to U.S. food aid products and programs.* Boston, MA, USA, Tufts University.

White, P.J. & Broadley, M.R. 2009. Biofortification of crops with seven mineral elements often lacking in human diets – iron, zinc, copper, calcium, magnesium, selenium and iodine. *New Phytologist*, 182(1): 49–84.

WHO (World Health Organization). 2000. *Obesity: preventing and managing the global epidemic.* WHO Technical Report Series No. 894. Geneva, Switzerland.

WHO. 2004. *Global Strategy on Diet, Physical Activity and Health*. Geneva, Switzerland.

WHO. 2008a. *The global burden of disease: 2004 update*. Geneva, Switzerland.

WHO. 2008b. *Worldwide prevalence of anaemia 1993–2005.* WHO Global Database on Anaemia. Geneva, Switzerland.

WHO. 2009a. *Global prevalence of vitamin A deficiency in population at risk 1995–2005.* WHO Global Database on Vitamin A Deficiency. Geneva, Switzerland.

WHO. 2010. *Set of recommendations on the marketing of foods and non-alcoholic beverages to children.* Geneva, Switzerland.

WHO. 2011a. *Global status report on noncommunicable diseases.* Geneva, Switzerland.

WHO. 2011b . *Nutrition-Friendly Schools Initiative (NFSI): a school-based programme to address the double burden of malnutrition.* Presentation (available at: www.who.int/nutrition/topics/NFSI_Briefing_presentation.pdf)

WHO. 2011c. *Regional Consultation on Food-Based Dietary Guidelines for countries in the Asia Region New Delhi, India, 6–9 December 2010. A report.* New Delhi. WHO Regional Office for South-East Asia.

WHO. 2013a. *Obesity and overweight.* Fact Sheet No. 311 (available at http://www.who.int/mediacentre/factsheets/fs311/en/).

WHO. 2013b. Global Database on Child Growth and Malnutrition (available at http://www.who.int/nutgrowthdb/about/introduction/en/index5.html).

WHO. 2013c. Global Health Observatory data repository. Risk factors: Overweight / Obesity (available at http://apps.who.int/gho/data/node.main.A896?lang=en).

WHO & FAO. 2003. *Diet, nutrition and the prevention of chronic diseases. Report of a Joint FAO/WHO Expert Consultation.* WHO Technical Report Series No. 916. Geneva, Switzerland.

Withrow, D. & Alter, D.A. 2010. The economic burden of obesity worldwide: a systematic review of the direct costs of obesity. *Obesity Reviews*, 12: 131–141.

Wojcicki, J.M. & Heyman, M.B. 2010. Malnutrition and the role of the soft drink industry in improving child health in sub-Saharan Africa. *Pediatrics*, 126(6): e1617–e1621.

World Bank. 2006a. *Repositioning nutrition as central to development: a strategy for large scale action.* Directions in Development. Washington, DC.

World Bank. 2006b. *Disease control priorities in developing countries*. Washington, DC.

World Bank. 2007a. *World Development Report 2008: Agriculture for development.* Washington, DC.

World Bank. 2007b. *From agriculture to nutrition: pathways, synergies and outcomes.* Report No. 40196-GLB. Washington, DC.

World Bank. 2008. *GDP per capita figures* (current US$). Webpage (available at http://data.worldbank.org/indicator/NY.GDP.PCAP.CD). Accessed 28 April 2012.

World Bank. 2011. *World Development Report 2012: Gender equality and development.* Washington, DC.

World Bank. 2013. *Improving nutrition through multisectoral approaches*. Washington, DC.

World Economic Forum. 2009. *The next billions: business strategies to enhance food value chains and empower the poor*. Geneva, Switzerland.

World Economic Forum. 2012. *The workplace wellness alliance investing in a sustainable workforce.* Geneva, Switzerland.

World Resources Institute in collaboration with UNEP, UNDP & World Bank. 1996. *World Resources Report 1996–97*. New York, USA, Oxford University Press.

Zameer, A. & Mukherjee, D. 2011. Food and grocery retail: patronage behavior of indian urban consumers. *South Asian Journal of Management*, 18(1): 119–134.

Special chapters of *The State of Food and Agriculture*

In addition to the usual review of the recent world food and agricultural situation, each issue of this report since 1957 has included one or more special studies on problems of longer-term interest. Special chapters in earlier issues have covered the following subjects:

1957 Factors influencing the trend of food consumption
Postwar changes in some institutional factors affecting agriculture
1958 Food and agricultural developments in Africa south of the Sahara
The growth of forest industries and their impact on the world's forests
1959 Agricultural incomes and levels of living in countries at different stages of economic development
Some general problems of agricultural development in less-developed countries in the light of postwar experience
1960 Programming for agricultural development
1961 Land reform and institutional change
Agricultural extension, education and research in Africa, Asia and Latin America
1962 The role of forest industries in the attack on economic underdevelopment
The livestock industry in less-developed countries
1963 Basic factors affecting the growth of productivity in agriculture
Fertilizer use: spearhead of agricultural development
1964 Protein nutrition: needs and prospects
Synthetics and their effects on agricultural trade
1966 Agriculture and industrialization
Rice in the world food economy
1967 Incentives and disincentives for farmers in developing countries
The management of fishery resources
1968 Raising agricultural productivity in developing countries through technological improvement
Improved storage and its contribution to world food supplies
1969 Agricultural marketing improvement programmes: some lessons from recent experience
Modernizing institutions to promote forestry development
1970 Agriculture at the threshold of the Second Development Decade
1971 Water pollution and its effects on living aquatic resources and fisheries
1972 Education and training for development
Accelerating agricultural research in the developing countries
1973 Agricultural employment in developing countries
1974 Population, food supply and agricultural development
1975 The Second United Nations Development Decade: mid-term review and appraisal
1976 Energy and agriculture
1977 The state of natural resources and the human environment for food and agriculture
1978 Problems and strategies in developing regions
1979 Forestry and rural development
1980 Marine fisheries in the new era of national jurisdiction
1981 Rural poverty in developing countries and means of poverty alleviation
1982 Livestock production: a world perspective
1983 Women in developing agriculture
1984 Urbanization, agriculture and food systems

1985	Energy use in agricultural production
	Environmental trends in food and agriculture
	Agricultural marketing and development
1986	Financing agricultural development
1987–88	Changing priorities for agricultural science and technology in developing countries
1989	Sustainable development and natural resource management
1990	Structural adjustment and agriculture
1991	Agricultural policies and issues: lessons from the 1980s and prospects for the 1990s
1992	Marine fisheries and the law of the sea: a decade of change
1993	Water policies and agriculture
1994	Forest development and policy dilemmas
1995	Agricultural trade: entering a new era?
1996	Food security: some macroeconomic dimensions
1997	The agroprocessing industry and economic development
1998	Rural non-farm income in developing countries
2000	World food and agriculture: lessons from the past 50 years
2001	Economic impacts of transboundary plant pests and animal diseases
2002	Agriculture and global public goods ten years after the Earth Summit
2003–04	Agricultural biotechnology: meeting the needs of the poor?
2005	Agriculture trade and poverty: can trade work for the poor?
2006	Food aid for food security?
2007	Paying farmers for environmental services
2008	Biofuels: prospects, risks and opportunities
2009	Livestock in the balance
2010–11	Women in agriculture: closing the gender gap for development
2012	Investing in agriculture for a better future